THE FOOD BABY DETOX

How to listen to your body:
discover the foods that cause tummy bloating,
food cravings, low energy & tank your sex drive.

Niki Driscoll, MS, HHP, LMT

ISBN-13: 978-1514841112
ISBN-10: 1514841118

No book can replace the services of a physician. Do not use any information
contained in this book to make a diagnosis, treat a health problem or replace your
doctor's advice. Bloating and other symptoms mentioned in this book may be the
cause of other more serious health conditions. Consult your physician before
beginning this and any diet program. Following recommendations does not ensure
that you will be healthy, as there are many factors that contribute to overall health.
The author hereby disclaims any and all liability resulting from injuries or damage
caused by following recommendations contained in this book.

To my darling children—who have taught me by example how to listen to my body and love my body.

CONTENTS

FOREWORD

Unlike real babies, you can show signs of a food baby after just one meal. But, the good news is that it doesn't take nine months to flatten a food baby tummy. The Food Baby Detox teaches you in 30 days how to self-discover the foods that are harming your body. It's the ultimate guide for following your gut instincts—your digestive gut and your intuitive gut.

Niki educates you on why you may ignore your gut and feel drawn towards no-good-for-you foods. She teaches you how to break the cycle of seeking these harmful foods—what she calls bad boyfriend foods. You know the foods that lie to you, manipulate how you feel and keep you coming back for more. No more! I might call them Prince Harming foods, based off my Oprah.com recommended book, *Prince Harming Syndrome*.

This is like a relationship book and a diet book all swirled together. Hello pure and good relationships—with your food, your body and yourself!

The core message is timeless—you must love yourself and trust yourself healthy!

Karen Salmansohn
Best-selling author of *How To Be Happy, Dammit!*, Founder of the Do-It Program

TERMS

Food Baby: Pregnant-like appearance caused from eating foods your body responds to negatively, including food sensitivity and food intolerance.

Gut: Sometimes used to refer to distended abdominals or abdominal fat. In the context of this book, 'gut' is a blanket term used to refer to the stomach, small intestine and large intestine.

Digestion: Digestion begins in the mouth, travels down the esophagus and ends up in the stomach, where food is digested and absorbed into the blood stream via digestive enzymes. Undigested food, waste and bacteria are moved into the large intestine for elimination.

Frenemy: A frenemy is a blend of friend and enemy.

A person with whom one is friendly despite a fundamental dislike or rivalry. ~Oxford Dictionary

The Food Baby Detox references 'bad' or 'harmful' bacteria as frenemy-bacteria because these bacteria do play a supportive role in digestion when properly balanced with the 'beneficial' or 'good' friendly-bacteria.

Detox: A process or period of time in which one abstains from or rids the body of toxic or unhealthy substances. ~Oxford Dictionary

Clean eating: Eating unprocessed foods found in nature that enhance a person's wellbeing. This excludes synthetic vitamins and compounds, genetically modified foods (GMO's), chemical additives, preservatives, emulsifiers or thickeners.

Paleo: A dietary philosophy rooted in eating what our paleolithic (cavemen) ancestors would have eaten. According to this dietary philosophy, our ancestors did not eat grains, legumes, potatoes or dairy. The Food Baby Detox is not a Paleo Diet, although it recognizes that a Paleo Diet is beneficial for some individuals. The Food Baby Detox believes in nutritional individuality and is founded on helping individuals self-discover what foods work for their unique bodies.

Nutritional Individuality: A dietary philosophy that believes each individual has a unique genetic requirement for food. There were different kinds of cave people based on the geographic availability of food. I like to call it 'Individualized Paleo.' This concept also goes by the name Biochemical Individuality, a term coined by Roger Williams and Metabolic Typing, as trademarked by the author of The Metabolic Typing Diet, William Wolcott.

Food Ratio: The relative amount of macronutrients (protein, fat and carbohydrates) consumed.

Mindset: The attitude, energy and outlook a person chooses. Mindset may be influenced by previous life experiences and programmed in the brain as a 'default' mode of behavior. However, mindset is mutable and within an individual's control to change with effort and awareness.

Toxin: A poisonous substance. The wrong food for your unique body can act like a poisonous substance.

HOW TO USE THIS BOOK

"You have to laugh at yourself because you'd cry your eyes out if you didn't" ~ The Indigo Girls

I know first hand how frustrating it can be to try every diet, health tip, gimmick and exercise available and still have a body that looks and feels unhealthy. Negative self talk, body bashing and poor health is serious. But too much seriousness is a buzz kill. So we're going to poke fun and laugh at food babies as we learn to heal them.

My intention for this book is to use nutrition as a self help tool to facilitate self exploration, reflection and ultimately mind-body reconnection.

You can't hate yourself healthy. Looking in the mirror and berating your body for not being enough will not motivate you to make healthier choices. Just like telling a kid that they're stupid doesn't motivate them to study more or strive for academic excellence. Kids who are told they are stupid—believe it. And if you falsely believe that you're fat, ugly, lazy or undisciplined, then you'll likely believe it, give up trying, or sabotage your best intentioned efforts. You must love yourself healthy by honoring your body as the container of who you really are, your spirit. Honor your own importance in the world by taking care of yourself with healthy choices.

THE BACKGROUND INFORMATION

The science behind food babies and abdominal bloating is presented in the first portion of this book. The Food Baby Detox aims to teach you how to intuitively listen to your body so you can determine your own needs. In order to learn to listen to your body, you need a fundamental understanding of how it works.

HOW TO TAKE ACTION

The second portion of the book lays out the step-by-step guidelines for The Food Baby Detox, including healing supplements, a healthy pantry guide and grocery lists to give you a baseline.

Knowing what to eat is only half of the equation. You have to be able transform the information into action—and feel good about it. Real results and true success occur when your body and mind are on the same page, mind-body connection. A body that needs kale but is thinking candy is in a state of mind-body disconnection.

In order to change your eating or self-talk habits, you have to be fully aware of what motivates and drives you. A great way to become aware is to capture your feelings on paper instead of allowing your innermost self to float through space—writing is a form of mind-body connection. At the end of each chapter you'll find self-reflective questions for your journaling pleasure.

Wishing you self-love and happiness,

Niki

WHAT IS A FOOD BABY?

The Food Baby has been around since the beginning of time, but became more prevalent in the early days of the millennium. The Oxford Dictionary added the term 'food baby' in 2013. Maybe the Oxford wordsmiths are getting hip to the times or maybe it's because the food baby is becoming so common it's worthy of its own modern definition.

Some food babies come and go. And others have chronic food babies.

You may have assumed food babies are the result of overeating, genetics or being overweight, however, the leading cause is something you may not have considered.

A food baby is a term used to describe abdominal bloating and distention that gives you a pregnant-like appearance. This happens from consuming foods that are not compatible with *your* body. The food baby is also referred to as a pouch, beer gut, or pot belly.

> *Foods that are not compatible with your body can be a food sensitivity, a food intolerance or the product of an unhealthy digestive system—all are addressed in The Food Baby Detox.*

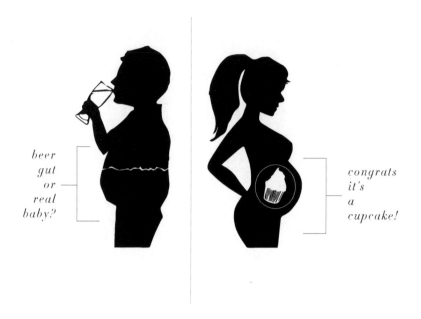

beer gut or real baby?

congrats it's a cupcake!

WHAT TO EXPECT WHEN YOU'RE EXPECTING

You've probably experienced the confusion between discerning a food baby belly and a real baby belly. They look so darn similar that they're hard to differentiate. Heck, I've experienced baby-daddy bewilderment about the origin of my own preggers belly. It's a tough call when both varieties of prego bellies look and feel the same.

Feeling unattractive and being the shamed mother of a bastard cheesecake isn't the only downside to a food baby. Food babies can be accompanied by other symptoms such as: back pain, headaches, skin problems, drippy nose, mucus in the throat, fluid retention and puffiness, mental fog, irritability, inability to fall asleep or stay asleep, weight gain and gas.

Maybe those symptoms don't sound like much to you. After all, no one ever died from having pimples, a post-nasal drip and impeccably timed flatulence. Unless, you're that person, I can tell you from first hand experience that being this person is soul-suffocating. I had a "food baby" for over ten years with zero results from the bazillions of crunches and countless hours of ab work that I did regularly. My concerned mother actually packed me copious amounts of Gas-X in my off-to-college care kit with instructions to take two prior to a date.

More serious food sensitivity symptoms include:
Irritable Bowel Syndrome, Migraine, Chronic Diarrhea, Heartburn/ GERD, Fibromyalgia, Arthritis, Joint Pain, Muscle Pain, Weight Imbalances, Chronic Fatigue, Chronic Sinusitis, Insomnia, Skin Eruptions, Autism/ADD.

> *Many symptoms that are characteristic of abdominal bloating and distention may also present in other pathologies such as: parasitic infection, fungal overgrowth, intestinal obstruction, tumor, heart failure, kidney disease, cirrhosis of the liver. The Food Baby Detox is not a cure all. If your symptoms improve and you look and feel better on The Food Baby Detox, then you have likely eliminated a food that is harmful for your body.*

A SELF DISCOVERY EXPERIMENT

At 23 years old, my health took a serious nosedive. I had a commercial-worthy list of symptoms including fatigue that caused me to sleep for an entire year! No exaggeration. I couldn't keep my eyes peeled open for more than two hours a day. I started doctor hopping to find out what the health was wrong with me! Diagnosis: depression. No duh, I was depressed! Who wants to be Sleeping Beauty with a chronic food baby? Not the most exciting Disney Princess. I knew depression was not the root cause of my health problems. I forced myself awake and started looking for my own answers.

At that time there was very little information about gut health, food sensitivities and intolerance. Through my research I discovered how to do an elimination diet to discover the foods that were harmful for my body. An elimination diet is an experimental break from any foods you suspect may be causing a negative response in your body. This break allows your body time to recover and heal. Once your food related symptoms have subsided, you experimentally add back one food at a time to see if you react to that food. The elimination diet that I did was very limited and impractical. Imagine eating nothing but lamb and pears for 3 weeks! Crazy. But don't worry, I created The Food Baby Detox as a practical elimination experiment, gut healing strategy and a way-of-life plan for keeping your health and hotness top notch without deprivation.

DO YOU LOVE INSTANT GRATIFICATION?

The New England Journal of Medicine debunked the myth that slow gradual changes create sustained long term weight loss. Just the opposite. The study found that people who experienced rapid weight loss in the initial phases were more likely to enjoy long term success. This is likely due to the fact that seeing a positive change is motivating.

Healing your gut and removing negative response foods from your day-to-day menu can give you fast results. Many of my clients lose up to ten pounds in the first week! One fine day in 2012, I ate a no-good-for-me food and a food baby was conceived. I followed The Food Baby Detox and eight days later I was sporting a flat tummy again. Below you'll see pictures of me pregnant (with a real baby in 2007), four hours after having a negative food response, followed by my progress four days and eight days later.

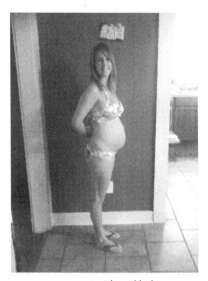

pregnant with real baby
(2007)

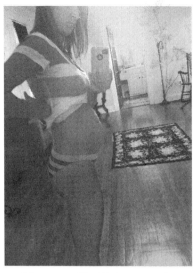

4 hours post food baby conception
(2012)

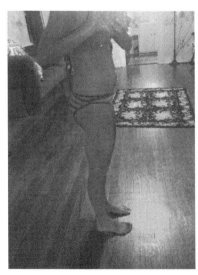

The Food Baby Detox day 4
(2012)

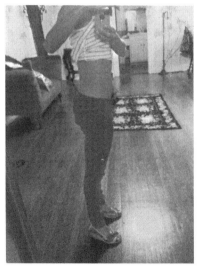

The Food Baby Detox day 8
(2012)

THE FOOD BABY PHENOMENON — EXPOSED

I know that food baby bloating can make you feel completely helpless when it comes to your body and health. You might feel like you've tried everything to get a flat stomach and lose abdominal fat. Eating low fat. Low carb. High protein. Counting calories. Exercising your ass off.

The good news is that you don't have to disavow (aka stop) eating fat, meat or even carbs. You don't have to starve yourself or count calories. It is within your power to control your health and achieve your ideal weight and body shape. You can do it by avoiding the foods that you do not digest well and are sensitive to. If you've had trouble flattening your tummy, losing weight, and finding a diet that works for you or if you feel the effects of sub-sparkly health, like low energy, flat sex drive or even bad skin; then it's likely you've wrangled with negative responses to the foods you are eating, including food intolerance and food sensitivity. You are not alone.

Populations across the globe are suffering from food babies and related symptoms. Recall, a food baby is the result of abdominal bloating and distention. Abdominal bloating has been defined as a subjective experience and sensation of abdominal swelling. Whereas, abdominal distention is a visible increase in abdominal girth. These symptoms have been almost exclusively studied in people with functional gastrointestinal (GI) disorders, which is the presence of GI symptoms that do not have an identifiable pathophysiology. Symptoms include bloating, distention, functional constipation and functional diarrhea. If you take a peek below at some formal definitions of functional bloating, constipation and diarrhea, you'll quickly realize that functional GI symptoms are routinely occurring in the general population. Plenty of people disregard food babies, constipation and diarrhea—not realizing that these symptoms are your body's way of saying something is not right.

I'm referencing Rome II Diagnostic Criteria for Functional

Gastrointestinal Disorders rather than the most recent version, Rome III, because the standards for diagnosis have been loosened. Some individuals who would have been diagnosed with a Functional Gastrointestinal Disorder under Rome II may be excluded when using Rome III Criteria. I believe the body speaks through symptoms to let us know our health is not on par. Symptoms are still meaningful even in the absence of an official diagnosis.

Functional Bloating, Constipation and Diarrhea must occur at least 12 weeks, which need not be consecutive, in the preceding 12 months:

Functional Bloating is a feeling of fullness, bloating, or visible distention and there is insufficient criteria for a diagnosis of functional dyspepsia, irritable bowel syndrome, or other functional disorder.

Functional Constipation includes two or more of the following symptoms occurring at least 25% of the time: straining, a sense of incomplete elimination, a sense of obstruction, the presence of hard to pass or lumpy stool, fewer than three bowel movements per week.

Functional Diarrhea is characterized by loose, mushy stools without abdominal pain or discomfort present 3/4 of the time.

In Chapter 6, we will talk more about what your bowel movements are supposed to look like, feel like and when they should occur.

The National Institute for Health (NIH) estimates that sixty to seventy million people suffer from functional gastrointestinal disorders. One study approximated that 96% of people with functional gastrointestinal disorders experience abdominal bloating with or without distention. A study from the American Journal of Gasteroenterology reported that bloating and distention were perceived as the most bothersome symptom in people with Functional GI disorders. Additionally, 10-30% of the general population (people who have not been diagnosed with a Functional GI disorder) also suffer from abdominal bloating and distention.

Population data based off of self-diagnostic (a.k.a. listen-to-your-body) questionnaires have shown symptoms of food intolerance (one of the causes of functional GI disorders) affects: forty five percent of Britain, thirty-three percent of Canadians, twenty to seventy-five percent of Australians and an estimated thirty percent of Americans. While these estimates are prone to criticism because of the subjectivity of the data, it demonstrates the large percentage of people who have an internal knowing that something is not right with their food choices and/or their digestion. Trust your gut!

A double-blind, placebo-controlled food challenge study published in the Lancet, estimated twenty percent of people in the UK have food intolerance. This particular study used eight foods in the food challenge. Several studies found the occurrence of food intolerance is higher in women.

Beyond the research and percentages, it's an observable fact that there is a cultural fear of saying, "congratulations!" or "when are you due?" It's taboo because your odds of being wrong are too high—keep your head down and your eyes to yourself. Unless, of course, you're criticizing a celebrity's body, then it's socially acceptable to call it like you see it. After all, everyone loves a good bump watch at someone else's expense. But, let us not forget, this uterus-confusion is not a female-specific problem. One summer afternoon by the pool, my then four year old son made the out loud observation, "I didn't know men could have babies." Sheesh kid, haven't you ever heard of a food baby?

The food baby phenomenon is growing in popularity among pop-cult sectors. There are entire photography and video collections of food babies across social media platforms including Tumblr, Instagram and Youtube. In 2012, I posted a free informational video on Youtube called

How to Get Rid of Your Food Baby. It sent food baby cult followers into a tizzy. The food baby cult followers seem to love their food babies and the self-jesting laughter that it provides them. Those that came across my YouTube video were vexed with me for providing a solution. One comment read, "You're a fraud. I wasted 5 minutes of my life before I figured out that you're trying to take my food baby away." "We love our food babies. Leave the food babies alone." Out of pure shock that people actually had endearment for their food babies, I removed the video. The food baby lovers inspired the sarcastic yet self-lovin' tone for this book.

SOCIAL ACCEPTANCE VS. SELF-ACCEPTANCE?

Maybe the food baby activists have it right. Should we simply self-accept and let it all hang out? Are we a superficial, shallow, body-obsessed culture for worrying about the size of our waistline? Have we been culturally indoctrinated to believe that flat-abs are sexy? Perhaps flat-abs are akin to the ancient Chinamen's foot fetish or the way Ethiopian men brazenly demand stretchy lips? And what about the cultures where overweight women are considered beautiful? How can we discern the difference between cultural beauty-brainwashing and our authentic aesthetic desires? How does health fit into this picture? And what does a healthy vibrant body look and feel like?

Do not dismiss the importance of feeling beautiful. It is important. But beyond looking good, there's health. Where do we draw the line between social aesthetic conformity and an aesthetic that represents a healthy vibrant body?

There are variances in the desired cultural aesthetic in the Western Hemisphere with preferences ranging from super model thin to an athletic figure. The Western culture seems to prefer a leaner and toned body regardless of structural build and body shape.

Generally speaking, there is nothing wrong with this preference. After all, we are not in famine, therefore there is no reason to hold excessive amounts of weight. We all understand the benefits of eating healthy and exercising regularly, both of which yield healthy body fat percentages and muscle tone. The problem lies in trying to stuff your unique body into a different mold. You won't ever achieve the super model thin mold if you're body type is prone to a higher (yet still healthy) body fat percentage, muscle mass and/or more curves. And sorry sister, if you are pin straight, you'll probably never look curvy and rubenesque. Let that be okay. The visual variety offered by different body types is a reason to celebrate. How creepy would life be if we were all clones from one mold? Men would be bored—not stiff.

Now, let's consider the cultures inclined to perceive heavier women as the gold standard for beauty, including some of the South Pacific Islands, Middle Eastern countries and African cultures. It's purported in the anthropological research that women from these areas have a genetic tendency to hold higher percentages of body fat as an evolutionary survival response to the feast-famine cycle inherent to the geography. A point of interest is that today some women in these cultures suffer with poor body image just like Western cultures. Many take extreme measures to gain weight including forcefully overeating and taking appetite stimulants. These cultures suffer from extremely high rates of obesity related disease and cardiovascular disease. The question: is the real issue social pressure to be thin-enough or fat-enough?

What if we (humans) dropped the motive of looking good and adopted the concept of feeling healthy? When you experience a life without health symptoms and you have tons of energy, your mentality can't help but change. Think back to a time when you were sick and exhausted. Wasn't it hard to feel happy and think clearly? That's because your physical body is linked to your emotional and mental state.

Vibrant health includes having emotional balance and mental clarity.

Make no mistake—your diet affects your biochemistry which affects your perception of yourself and the world around you. Let's consider that body image distortion is a byproduct of unclear thinking and faulty perception of oneself. Is it possible that if each of us chose nourishing foods for our unique bodies we might improve our entire being and outlook, body-mind-spirit?

The New England Journal of Medicine thinks the mind-body connection is impacted by food. They linked a myriad of psychiatric conditions such as anxiety and depression as being caused by gluten intolerance!

Dr. Natasha Campbell-McBride's research also presents compelling evidence for the mind-body connection. In her book, Gut and Psychology Syndrome, she describes the chemical process and effect on perception that results from the presence of negative food responses. Certain foods will actually ferment inside of an unhealthy gut and create an alcohol. As most of us have experienced, alcohol moves through the gut and goes directly into the bloodstream with near immediate affects on the brain and perception. What I'm saying is that if your digestive system is unhealthy or your food choices aren't right for your body, it is possible to experience a chronic low level intoxication from the foods you are eating, which will absolutely affect your mood, attitude and perception!

When you nourish and support your body with healthy choices, you naturally radiate your inherent beauty, inside and out. And we were all designed to be healthy and beautiful.

Despite the odd cultural particulars of thin, fat and fetish driven aesthetic goals, from an evolutionary psychology perspective, all species have a natural sexual attraction to a physical build that represents healthy. Humans have a primal center in the brain, called the reptilian brain, which contains ancestral data for natural and sexual selection for survival. Survivalist theorists, such as Darwin and his post-modern proteges, suggest that the primal brain processes and interprets an unhealthy appearance as a threat to species perpetuation.

Notwithstanding genetic variance, social and personal preference, there does appear to be some congruency in cross-cultural standards of beauty that represent a healthy body, including clear skin, overall body symmetry and proportion. One of the pioneers in evolutionary psychology, Devendra Singh, theorized that women with a low waist to hip ratio (WHR) are considered more attractive cross-culturally, regardless of structural build and body fat percentage. This means that the relative proportion of fat distribution is less in the waist and more in the hips. In fact, it is medically accepted that having an unhealthy waist to hip ratio is a predictive factor for diabetes, cancer and premature death from cardiovascular disease.

Take a look at each of the women in the lineup on the next page. Each woman has a vastly different body type, yet all have a healthy WHR.

The WHR measurement was intended to be predictive of fat distribution, specifically abdominal fat. This measurement does not account for the presence of bloating and/or distention which may also significantly contribute to an increase in waist line circumference. Although there is an absence of literature on the subject, I consider it highly possible — if not likely, that a high WHR may be additionally influenced to a large degree by abdominal bloating and distention, in addition to actual abdominal fat. The limitations of the WHR as a sole indicator for the intention of measuring abdominal fat is a philosophical presupposition. Nonetheless, the measurement still holds a significant predictive value for determining overall health and in turn, perceived attractiveness. In fact, food baby bloating and distention increases the waist line.

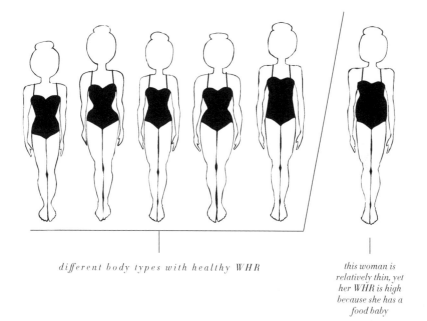

different body types with healthy WHR

this woman is relatively thin, yet her WHR is high because she has a food baby

The visual appearance of a swollen, food baby belly is likely interpreted (by you and others) as unhealthy—because it is. Feeling unattractive about your food baby may be explained by evolutionary psychology operating in your subconscious mind as a way to communicate to you that your health is not up-to-par! Your feelings are health warnings saying "Hey, you have a food-induced pregnancy and that's not normal or healthy!"

Your food baby is harming more than your bikini body. It's harming your health. Food babies are a common symptom of food sensitivity and intolerance. To be clear, a symptom is a sign or indication that a deeper problem or imbalance is present. Symptoms are gentle communications from your body to let you know that your health is dis-easy. In other words, on the road to disease—if something doesn't change. It's like a warning light in your car. Most of the time you can drive around with the light on for a long time before the car breaks down. However,

13

responsible and respectful owners of vehicles take care of problems proactively — before a 'breakdown' occurs. Dis-easy health complaints related to negative food responses that you may struggle with include weight problems, low energy and fatigue, low sex drive, problematic skin, digestive problems, headaches or food cravings. These symptoms aren't bad. They're actually very helpful if you understand what your body is trying to communicate to you. Throughout The Food Baby Detox, you will learn how to listen to your body and love it for being an effective communicator.

IT'S EASIER TO LOVE YOUR BODY — WHEN YOU UNDERSTAND IT

Despite your food baby challenge, you should extend love to yourself; food baby, fat rolls, potty problems and all. Be grateful to your body for being a good-damn warrior. Your body has adapted to this modern junk food saturated world with grace (and baby doll fashion t-shirts). You're still here and you're still kicking. That's something to be proud of. So, hell yes and mad props for self-love!

But, hell no for settling! You are not a body-obsessed, control-freak-perfectionist for being dissatisfied with your food baby. Your dissatisfaction means you know on a 'gut' level that something is not right. Don't ignore that uneasiness you feel. That's your true desire, it's your soul trying to bust out of your body cage. Your body will limit you with symptoms as a way to detain you from continuing on your current path. To be set free of symptoms you have to listen to your body. You have to live your entire life inside of your body, you may as well get along with it.

MAKE SELF-LOVE NOT SELF-WAR

It's self-loving to take action in healing your body. Because you can't float off into the wild blue yonder if you're wander lusting for a coverup, a toilet, an aspirin or a nap. Your free spirit was designed to live in a symptom-free body. Free-spirit 101 tells us that we should always validate our own internal knowing. No one knows you better than you. You don't need a doctor to tell you that food baby bloating and distention isn't healthy. You already know it's not healthy because it feels terrible—heavy, tired, gassy, backed-up, crampy, constipated or it instigates an urge-to-purge, one way or another.

You've probably tried different ways of getting rid of your food baby like:
• eating smaller portions or starving yourself
• counting calories
• consuming whole foods
• abdominal exercises, cardio, cross fit, yoga and every fitness craze in between
• collecting diet books and exercise magazines

I'm not dogging these methods for getting healthy or losing weight because clearly overeating, junk food and lack of exercise is a recipe for weight gain and an unshapely body. But with a food baby, you can do crunches all day long and still not achieve the results you are truly looking for because your abdominal muscles are not the problem. You can cut calories and lose weight, body fat is not the problem. The problem is what you put into your body and what is causing you to bloat, hold excess weight, retain water, create skin problems, food cravings and crash your sex drive.

Unfortunately in health we do not get an 'A' for effort. That's a frustrating truth when you've proven yourself with 'A' worthy efforts, discipline and perseverance.

The reality is your food baby will not disappear until you remove the intolerant foods from your diet and replace them with healing foods and supplements. The good news is, you may just look and feel significantly better within the first week of the The Food Baby Detox!

THE FOOD BABY DETOX IS A NUTRITIONAL GUIDE FOR LIFE

The Food Baby Detox is different from other detoxes. Most traditional detoxes cleanse your body of toxins over a specified period of time. However, most fail to address the reason why our bodies are overburdened to begin with and as soon as the detox is over, people head for their old (often toxic) foods again. The primary source of toxins is never addressed and the effects of the detox are marginal at best.

> *A detox is a method of removing harmful or toxic substances from the body. The Food Baby Detox is a customized detox that frees you from harmful or toxic foods for your unique body.*

The Food Baby Detox is a self-discovery experiment and a lesson in listening to your body. When you develop a relationship with your body you can detect the subtle symptoms and toxic effects that occur from eating the wrong foods in the wrong amounts *for you*. You will also discover what foods make you feel amazing! After a while, choosing *your* compatible foods becomes an intuitive process.

This detox begins by guiding you to identify what foods in your diet are creating toxic reactions. We all have food issues. You do. I do. Toxic overload from food is a modern day problem. There are certain foods that are universally toxic like donuts, fried chicken and gummy worms. But, the kicker is that many of the foods that you might think are healthy may not be healthy for YOU.

Food provides information to your body. Information is power. Food has the power to vitalize you and build you stronger. It also has the power to break you down and zap you. This is nothing new. Roman poet, Lucretius pegged this concept in his circa 99-55 B.C. quote, "One man's food is another man's poison." In other words, food alters your biochemistry for better or for worse.

The Food Baby Detox is a 30 day experimental elimination of the most common foods that cause negative responses, including food intolerance and food sensitivity. We'll call them the Top Eight culprit foods.

Processed Foods   Sugar/Artifical Sugar   Soy   Gluten   Dairy   Eggs   Corn   Legumes

You may feel overwhelmed at the idea of eliminating these foods. That's perfectly normal. Remind yourself, The Food Baby Detox is only 30 days. You can do this! Because it's not a promise to never-ever have these foods again. This is not a break-up with the Top Eight foods, just a break. Tell your Top Eight foods, "It's not you, it's me. I need some time alone to figure things out."

Freedom from these foods gives your body time and space to heal. After 30 days on The Food Baby Detox you will reintroduce one food at a time to determine whether you are reactive to that food. You may discover that you're A-okay on some foods. If you are still reactive, you'll feel the effects of the reintroduced food. At that point you may need to re-free yourself from the food for a longer time period like 60 or 90 days, up to a full year.

The elimination period can vary by person, depending on how long you've had symptoms. When you realize how bad a particular food makes you look and feel, you'll find it easier to be free of it. One of the most common things I hear from my clients is how they didn't realize how unmotivated, lethargic and self-destructive they felt while consuming the Top Eight foods until they discovered how pure, clear, energetic and productive they feel when free of negative food responses.

If you've consumed the Top Eight foods your whole life, you likely have no reference point for what being free of these foods feels like. It's possible that you feel like rubbish and don't even realize it! You may think that's just the way your body is or that it's genetic.

YOU ARE MEANT TO BE HEALTHY — IT'S IN THE HUMAN DESIGN

Dr. Weston A Price (1870-1948) presents compelling evidence in his research that demonstrates human health as a birthright rather than a genetic stroke of luck. He documented in his book, *Nutrition and Physical Degeneration*, his examination of over 30 tribes from around the world who were eating their native diets and had not yet been exposed to modern food processing. His research revealed that there was very little incidence of disease among the tribes who ate their native diets. However, the younger generations who were exposed to and ate modern processed food were frequently subject to tooth decay, degenerative disease, allergies, arthritis, diabetes, intestinal complaints and chronic fatigue just to name a few.

WHAT IS HEALTHY?

Truly healthy people are few and far between. The National Institute of Health estimates that nearly 70% of the US population is overweight or obese and 80% of people have suffered acne at some point in their lives. According to a study published in Behavioral Medicine, fatigue is ranked as one of the leading health complaints among teenagers and young adults. Roughly 15% of the population has an IBS diagnosis and another 15% are constipated. One study found that 32% of women and 15% of men have Hypoactive Sexual Desire Disorder (HSDD), the lack or absence of sexual desire. I wish that was a joke. Seriously, that statistic only includes individuals who meet the clinical criteria for low sex drive. I suspect most people with low sex drives aren't scheduling appointments to say, "Doc, I'm not horny." Most of us push symptoms like that to the back burner and drudge on.

ILL-HEALTH IS NOT THE NEW NORMAL

It seems everyone has something out-of-whack. But, it is not normal to have a food baby, to be overweight, to have low energy, bad skin, insatiable cravings for unhealthy foods or a low sex drive.

A DAY IN THE LIFE OF 'REAL' NORMAL

Normal health is supposed to go like this: You fall asleep easily, you stay asleep and wake up feeling rested after 7-9 hours of sleep. Your metabolism is revved and ready to go. Your breakfast balances and fuels you with the energy, an emotional uplift and the mental clarity to sustain you until the next meal. No need to snack. No cravings. No energy dips. Just clear thinking, focus and pep in your step. Each meal of the day provides your body with positive feedback like remaining the same size jeans before and after eating. At some point during the day you feel an urge to express yourself through movement. It will be a nonnegotiable need and a pleasure, not a should or have-to. Speaking of non-negotiable urges, you'll also need to eliminate your bowels. There isn't a do-it-later option like procrastinating laundry duty. It also shouldn't be like a football player rushing the field. It should be more casual, in a it's-time-to-powder-my-nose manner of grace. (In Chapter 5, we'll talk more about how your potty piece de resistance is actually telling you what to eat and what not to eat.) At the end of your 'normal' day, you take off your fancy frocks and you still look like a trendsetter without a stitch. Your well-shaped body is cloaked in clear bright skin and you have a soulful gleam in your eye. You are boundless and up for anything. Hobbies. Hanging out. Sex. A dance party in your nighties. Whatever. You're game.

This vision is not unrealistic. It is what's possible if you choose to self-discover on The Food Baby Detox. You can live the dream.

LET'S ADDRESS THE INITIAL SHOCK, SOME OF THE FOODS THAT GIVE YOU RESPITE DURING YOUR DAY ARE KEEPING YOU FROM YOUR FULL POTENTIAL

I'll never forget the day I was advised to quit eating gluten and dairy containing foods. I had an instinctive middle finger reaction. What the *health* was I supposed to eat? I felt baffled trying to imagine what to put on my empty plate. Was life worth living without gluten-stuffed scones and dairy-drenched cappuccinos? It turns out that I've got the drama queen gene. It wasn't as hard as I thought. If it was awful, I wouldn't do it. I do not believe that your eating-style should control your lifestyle because food is supposed to be pleasurable, even foodgasmic. I do not believe you have to feel like a junk-food junkie in withdrawal. Feeling deprived is not okay with me. What's the point of having a good-looking body if you feel empty?

YOUR WALLET DOESN'T HAVE TO BE EMPTIED EITHER

You can do The Food Baby Detox on a budget, while traveling and without eating anything weird. I'll show you a how-to with grocery lists, pantry guides and a packing-for-travel guide in Chapters 6 and 7. A tough aspect of starting a new routine in life is the inability to imagine what it looks like in your head. That's why The Food Baby Detox takes the guesswork out of your equation. All you have to do is follow the step by step process. Voila! You and The Food Baby Detox equal the ultimate makeover for your body and your life. You can change your body shape, lose weight, clear up your skin, get rid of your food cravings, improve your sex life and have amazing energy!

Here's a snapshot of what we'll be talking about in the upcoming chapters:

Step 1.
Experimentally Eliminate

Processed Foods   Sugar/Artifical Sugar   Soy   Gluten   Dairy   Eggs   Corn   Legumes

The simplest way to determine if you're having a negative response to any of the Top Eight intolerant foods is to eliminate them from your diet and monitor how you feel when you're off of those foods. If your stomach flattens, you lose weight, you experience an increase in energy or sex drive, your skin clears and your food cravings decrease, then it's likely that you eliminated a food that wasn't compatible with your body. It's important to remember that this is an experiment and it's only for 30 days! You have no way of knowing whether these foods are good or bad for you unless you try the experimental elimination. During the elimination, you can still enjoy flavorful food and the experience of eating.

Step 2.
Rotate Your Foods

A huge reason for the development of food intolerance is the overconsumption of the same foods day in and day out. The Top Eight foods are consumed frequently and in a lot of cases daily. Rotating your foods means ensuring that you are not eating the same foods every day. This prevents other food intolerance from developing, allows your body to receive a variety of nutrients needed for great health and it prevents culinary boredom and cravings. Mix things up and diversify your daily plate.

Step 3.
Reintroduce

Fermented Soy   Gluten   Dairy   Eggs   Corn   Legumes

At the end of 30 days you will reintroduce one culprit food at time excluding processed foods, sugar and artificial sugar - these foods aren't good for anyone and should rarely be consumed. This is not a junk food permission slip. This is a time to gather information about what works for your unique body or what doesn't work for you. Aren't you fed up with constantly searching for the next best diet? Aren't you ready to feed and satisfy your body? One thing is for certain, your body will not function at its best (which also means looking its best) when you feed it junk. The reintroduction phase is to determine your reaction to these foods in their healthy, whole food form.

Step 4.
Connect and Heal

The Food Baby Detox is a self-discovery process to determine your culprit foods. But really, it's a process of nourishing your self-connection to your body. A large part of not knowing what to eat is not knowing how to listen to your body. Your body reacts every time you eat. Ideally you should have a renewed sense of energy, mental clarity and emotional balance. Cravings are a sign that something is missing in your nutrition or your relationship with food. Explore yourself through self-reflection and answering the questions at the end of each chapter to build a full-filling relationship with food. The point of eating healthy is to allow you to live more, not less. Chapter 6 includes further insight into how your body gives you feedback about the foods you've eaten (it talks to you in the bathroom) and provides supplement recommendations to encourage the healing of your digestion.

Step 5.
The Food Baby Detox for Life!

The Food Baby Detox isn't a one-time experiment. You and your body are constantly changing. This includes what your body needs nutritionally. I recommend checking-in with your body's response to every meal. Take a moment to slow down. Enjoy your food. Feel your body. And respect what your body says to you. Your relationship with your food and your body require constant nurturing. I also recommend doing an annual reassessment of your needs using the principles in The Food Baby Detox.

THE FOOD BABY DETOX RESULTS

Case Study: Brittany, age 35, Attorney

I had struggled with my weight since I was a child. When I was 24, I decided to do something about it. I ran a couple of marathons and ate healthy yet I was still overweight, felt frustrated, discouraged and lacked confidence in myself. Fashion and shopping is my passion and an artistic expression of who I am. Since I lacked confidence, fashion became a method of hiding rather than expressing. I was willing to try anything and what Niki said made sense. I eliminated the foods I was intolerant to and my weight finally balanced! I threw out my size 14 wardrobe and celebrated in my new size 6 fashion. I fell asleep faster, felt rested in the morning and I suddenly felt excited about my life. Best of all, I don't have to starve or kill myself at the gym, because I know how to work with, rather than against my body.

Case Study: Greg, age 38, Actor

I've never been overweight but no matter what I've never been able to lose that last layer of fat around my midsection. I was weight training 5 times per week and doing cardio. I was feeling fed up and willing to try anything. Luckily, I met Niki and she encouraged me to try The Food Baby Detox. The best part about working with Niki was that she combines her knowledge of fat loss within The Food Baby Detox. After 6 days, my abs flattened and I became significantly leaner. After 3 weeks, I had gained a lot more muscle, lost my love handles and my 'puffy' appearance. My energy levels increased. My thought processes became more clear and focused. When I started the program I was just doing it to look better but the real bonus is that I have boatloads of energy and motivation. Now, if I eat something that my body doesn't like, my body actually feels hung over afterwards. Cleaning up your body makes your body more sensitive. No kidding. With food hangovers as a consequence, I find it real easy to stick to foods that are good for me.

Hanna, age 35, Real Estate Agent

Before I started The Food Baby Detox, I thought I was doing the right thing for my body as far as dieting. I thought that by eating very low fat that I would be thin and toned. I was working out very hard but not seeing any improvement. My diet consisted of protein shakes, protein bars, grilled chicken and veggies for lunch and a salad or vegetables for dinner. I have a sweet tooth and I was eating tiny nibbles of things like gummy bears, lemon heads and other candies when I got the urge to eat something sweet. When Niki presented her Food Baby Detox meal plan to me I was very nervous. On the detox I learned that "fat is your friend" when I had previously believed that fat was the enemy. I was overwhelmed by the amount of food that she was telling me to consume on a daily basis and was terrified that I was going to gain weight. I didn't understand that I could have a good body and feel satisfied at the same time. I had nothing to lose and kept telling myself that I had to trust The Food Baby Detox. I gave it a shot. The biggest change I noticed in those first few days was my energy levels. I had more energy and I physically felt stronger. The intolerant food including the sugar I was eating was weighing me down in the afternoon. Once I stopped eating it, I wasn't tired anymore. Now, I feel great physically and emotionally. My problem areas aren't problems anymore! I'm looking forward to continuing on The Food Baby Detox journey as a way of life!

introduction

SELF-REFLECTIVE JOURNAL

———

Take Your Before Picture: Inside and Out

It's great to get a baseline assessment for where you currently are with your health, body image and mentality, before you start The Food Baby Detox. I recommend taking the self-assessment below and taking a before picture. You can use your before picture as future inspiration. When you're scampering around proud of your effort and accomplishment, you will value this as reminder to yourself about how you are strong, committed and worth the effort.

What areas of your health would you like to improve?
- [ ] cravings
- [ ] body image and self-talk
- [ ] physical energy
- [ ] think more clearly
- [ ] weight loss
- [ ] improve body shape
- [ ] clear complexion
- [ ] knowledge about nutrition
- [ ] follow through and commitment to my health
- [ ] energy levels
- [ ] pace of living
- [ ] support system

What's your biggest block towards eating healthy?
- ☐ lack of knowledge
- ☐ lack of motivation
- ☐ lack of time
- ☐ lack of support
- ☐ lack of energy
- ☐ lack of feeling worth it
- ☐ lack of cooking skills

• What would happen if you continued on your current path?

Good news! The Food Baby Detox addresses all of your above concerns!

chapter one

WHAT CAUSES A FOOD BABY?

———

FOOD BABY FASHION, FRIENDS AND FRENEMIES

I had a food baby from the time I was 6 years old until I was in my late twenties. Hiding my body was constantly on my mind. My food baby followed me on every shopping expedition, gymnastics class and pool party. Most people probably thought of me as a bit of a fashionista because most days I wore a dress. What they didn't know is that I preferred dresses because they didn't cinch my tummy and cause discomfort. Best of all flowy dresses hid my food baby.

Wearing dresses wasn't my only food baby trick. I also discovered that I had a flatter tummy in the morning and by lunch I was back to sporting maternity clothes. This discovery led me to the false conclusion that restricting my overall food intake would make my stomach flat. But no matter how thin I became my food baby bloating remained because I was still eating the same foods that caused the problem. The next strategy I tried was not eating — at all. And guess what? It worked. The food baby disappeared because I was avoiding the foods that weren't right for my body. Obviously, anorexia is not the answer. I just traded one problem for a laundry list of other problems. But the point is that I was trying to listen to my body the best way I knew how.

It seems that I'm not alone with this experience. The International

Journal of Eating Disorders published a case history of a woman presenting with restrictive eating patterns and body dissatisfaction. This publication warned against misdiagnosis of anorexia nervosa in cases where bloating is a primary complaint as this may be indicative of a negative food response. In this case, the food aversion was instinctual and self-preserving due to the fact that the woman had celiac disease (gluten allergy).

THE FOOD BABY UNCOVERED

It's pretty clear that there's a correlation between what you eat and the conception of a food baby. Most people believe that a food baby is the natural consequence of overeating or a genetic misfortune.

There is a normal expansion of the stomach as it's filled with food and water. It is also normal to have fluctuations in the appearance of your abs throughout the day due to variances in your sodium intake and your hydration levels which influence the amount of water your body holds. But normal expansion doesn't cause discomfort, bloating or a significant increase in waist circumference, known as distention. A food baby is not a normal consequence of drinking, eating or overeating. A food baby is a response from drinking or eating a sensitive food, intolerant food, or a food that you do not digest well.

In some cases, a food baby can be created from less than 1 gram of a food you are sensitive to. A food baby is not an exclusive problem for junk food junkies, although consistently eating junk food is one way a food baby can occur. Food babies can also be caused by healthy foods. Any food, food additive, herb or spice can create a food baby if your body is sensitive, intolerant or doesn't have the ability to properly digest it. While any food can be the culprit, the following foods are the Top Eight culprits for negative food responses.

Processed Foods   Sugar/Artifical Sugar   Soy   Gluten   Dairy   Eggs   Corn   Legumes

These foods commonly elicit an inflammatory response that specifically affects the inside of the gut. Gut inflammation, like any inflammation, is characterized by redness, heat, pain and swelling. Internal inflammation and swelling poufs out the abdominal wall which creates the distended appearance characteristic of a food baby. A food baby is the product of gut inflammation.

YOU MIGHT BE WONDERING WHAT THE DIFFERENCE IS BETWEEN A FOOD ALLERGY, FOOD SENSITIVITY AND A FOOD INTOLERANCE

Food allergies trigger immediate and aggressive reactions in the immune system and are characterized by specific markers, called antigens, which are used by the body to identify foreign invaders, in this case food. Immunoglobulin E, IgE is the antibody response that occurs with allergies and is characterized by a swift histamine response causing swelling, itching, rash, nausea, shortness of breath, diarrhea and stomach pain. Most people know about the dangers of food allergies and people who have them are typically privy to their existence. But most people do not know about food sensitivity and intolerance.

Food sensitivity, often confused with and used interchangeably to describe food intolerance, is a non-allergic food hypersensitivity invoking inflammation and thereby an indirect immune response. Symptoms of food sensitivity manifest far more slowly than symptoms of a food allergy. Following exposure, symptoms can occur anywhere from several hours to a few days after eating an offensive food. The delayed symptom-response time makes it difficult to connect the dots between a food sensitivity and the related symptoms. Would you believe a food you ate three days ago caused your headache or broken-out skin today? What if you ate the same sensitive foods every day or nearly every day? What if you ate more than one sensitive food at the same time? Most people do. Research shows that the average person routinely eats the same 10-12 foods throughout their entire life. That's a no-go for the body. Your body needs healing time away from each particular food that you consume, even foods you tolerate well. We'll talk more about how to give your body a healing break in Chapter 5.

Food intolerance is the inability to digest certain foods due to a lack of digestive enzymes needed to break down that food. Enzyme deficiencies are commonly acquired due to our modern lifestyles. Food intolerance can alter the environment of your digestive system making you prone to develop food sensitivities and vice versa.

The common denominator for both food intolerance and food sensitivities is that they both create inflammation in the body, which we will describe in more detail in a bit. In the context of The Food Baby Detox, it is immaterial to define whether you have a food intolerance or a food sensitivity, both are negative food responses.

The whole fabulous point of The Food Baby Detox is to develop a relationship with your body to self-discover what works for you and what doesn't. From here on out we will refer (interchangeably) to a negative personal response to food as an intolerant food, Top Eight food or a culprit food.

DIFFERENT STROKES FOR DIFFERENT FOLKS

The Food Baby Detox is not a diet, a trend or a one size fits all approach to healing. Everyone has a unique body and biochemistry which will cause them to respond to food differently. Your body gives you feedback about your food choices through your energy levels, physical symptoms and through the clarity of your mental processes. Foods that create a significant amount of stress and inflammation inside of your body distort your body's feedback to you. My dad used to tell me the quickest remedy for an ache or a pain is to slam your hand in the door. Clearly, he has a dry sense of humor. But the point is, immediate pain trumps your ability to feel more subtle nuances. Food intolerance is like your hand slammed in the door. The immediate pain-sensations from bloating, fatigue and mental distraction about how you look and feel trump the subtle messages your body sends you about what to eat and not to eat. The Food Baby Detox eliminates the most common culprit foods to cleanse your body of the negative food responses so you can feel and acknowledge what your body is saying to you about what it really needs. It's a process of self-discovery.

Some people will discover that they can tolerate certain foods after a healing break from that food. Others will discover that they have a genetic intolerance, meaning their bodies weren't designed to ever tolerate a specific food.

As an example, a study published in the Journal of Gasteroenterology found that people of African and Asian decent are less likely to produce lactase, the enzyme that breaks down lactose, a sugar found in dairy products. In order to survive the cold climate, people of northern European descent genetically adapted to produce more lactase because they relied on dairy when crops weren't viable. Anthropological data suggests that grains originated in the Middle East about 10,000 years ago allowing people of that descent a better ability to digest the proteins, gluten and gliadin, found in grains. One study analyzed the genetic markers for celiac disease (an allergy to gluten) in the skeleton of an Italian woman dating back to the first century. The analysis determined that the woman was likely suffering from malnutrition due to celiac disease, which suggests she had a genetic predisposition towards a negative food response to grain proteins. Current research shows that the most common occurrence of celiac disease as well as gluten intolerance occur in people of European descent. I'm not saying that every Asian will be lactose intolerant. Nor am I saying that if you're not Asian you should celebrate your race with a cheese party. Ditto for the gluten statistics. I'm just conveying that genetics plays a role in how your body responds to food.

THE FOOD BABY ULTRASOUND - DISCOVER WHAT'S GOING ON - ON THE INSIDE

1. Your mouth is a portal for many microorganisms, chemicals and toxins to enter your body.

2. We survive thanks to the friendly bacteria that line the entire length of the digestive tract. These devoted friends create a buffer between your gut wall and any pathogens that creep in.

3. Your gut also has bacteria that protect your body by chelating toxins and heavy metals, absorbing carcinogenic substances and protecting against undigested food particles. They give the 411 to your immune system to create the production of natural antibiotic, antiviral and antifungal-like substances as a safeguard against pathogens.

4. You also have bad bacteria in your gut. Because these bacteria do add value to your life by assisting with the digestion of food, we'll call them frenemy bacteria, a blend between a friend and an enemy. There's nothing wrong with having a few frenemy bacteria as long as you keep the numbers low. Fortunately, if you have enough friendly bacteria, they will protect you by producing organic acids that lower pH and make your gut wall environment too acidic for frenemy bacteria overgrowth. This keeps the frenemy bacteria population in check. Beware—your frenemy bacteria are constantly looking for an opportunity to take over. But, you have more control than you think. Your lifestyle and food choices dictate how many friends and frenemies you make.

Here are some of the most common ways that friend-to-frenemy (good to bad) bacterial ratios can become imbalanced.

Antibiotics	Birth Control Pills
NSAIDS (ibuprofen and aspirin)	Junk Food
Steroid Drugs like Prednisolone, Hydrocortisone	Food Intolerance
Disease and Infections	Stress

Ideally you want your friend-to-frenemy bacterial ratio to be 85% friendly to 15% frenemy. Research shows that the friend-to-frenemy ratio is flipped in most people! Unfortunately, when you have accumulated a lot of frenemy bacteria, changing your eating habits alone is not always enough to escape the gut-damage from your past. In Chapter 6 of The Food Baby Detox you will get a supplement plan for healing your digestion and balancing your gut bacterial ratios. You can also visit nikidriscoll.com/foodbabydetoxsupplements for more information.

Your body's first line of defense from pathogens (such as bacteria and viruses) is a lining that runs from your mouth to your anus. This lining, called the mucosal barrier, comprises 80% of your immune system and is a major player in digestion. The intestinal mucosal barrier contains finger-like structures called villi. The villi surface is lined with cells that release digestive enzymes, absorb food and allow nutrients into the bloodstream. These cells are called enterocytes.

Enterocytes have an uncanny resemblance to the furry haired doll, Trolls. Your friendly bacterial flora plays a huge role in keeping your Trolls hair healthy. And we all know how important healthy hair is.

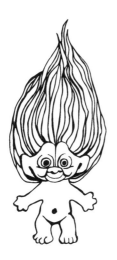

This luscious thick head of digestive-enzyme-releasing hair is the result of a healthy gut bacterial ratio. The thick hair acts to catch and absorb food particles/ nutrients.

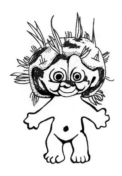

This Rogaine-needy, bald head is the result of unhealthy gut bacterial ratios, also known as gut dysbiosis. Without thick hair, even the best foods can't be absorbed and food particles go undigested. Undigested food particles rot, ferment and trigger an immune response and inflammation.

A healthy gut should be full of good-bacteria and 'hairy' enterocytes. The accumulation of too many frenemy bacteria damages the enterocytes and prevents them from properly digesting food. This results in gut inflammation, swelling and expansion that allows microorganisms, toxins, waste and undigested food particles to leak out of the gut. This is called Leaky Gut Syndrome. Food has no business being outside the gut wall so your body creates an indirect immune response (antigen formation) against that food—a food sensitivity.

Every time you eat an inflammatory food your body elicits an immune response that creates inflammation. This internal inflammation in the gut pushes the abdominal wall out and you get a food baby, a pouch or a potbelly.

Modern lifestyle choices such as food ruts, junk food and alcohol are large contributors to gut inflammation and food baby related symptoms.

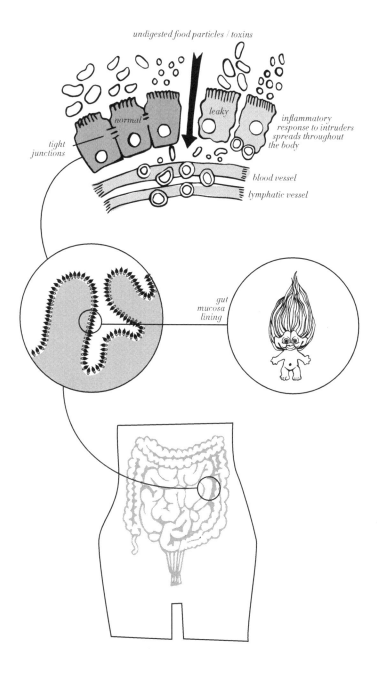

FOOD RUTS

Our lives are busy-busy-busy. We rush out in the morning, work through lunch and get home late. We drive through and roll on. If we do happen to hit the grocery store we tend to reach for the same old things. As mentioned earlier, most people's diet is composed of the same 12 foods their whole lives! This lack of nutritional variety is a major contributor to food sensitivity. What's more depraved than limiting yourself to the same cuisine day in and day out? Get ready to spice things up with some variety!

JUNK FOOD

Highly processed and refined foods, better known as junk food, commonly include the Top Eight intolerant foods as ingredients. The overuse of these ingredients burdens our digestive system and our bodies never get a break. Even worse than that, junk foods contain nutrient-deficient versions of the Top Eight intolerant foods including refined sugar, artificial sweeteners, high fructose corn syrup and processed soy. Unfortunately, many of these foods are marketed as healthy or labelled with the word 'free' (gluten-free, dairy-free, soy-free, sugar-free), yet these are actually junk foods in disguise. Energy bars, soy milk, protein powders and salad dressings are great hiding places for the Top Eight intolerant foods (see Chapter 3 for more information).

Imagine if you ate the same offending foods or food additives frequently, then you may become chronically inflamed and acquire a chronic first trimester like appearance. In other words, food intolerance can create a food baby that always stays with you. A beer gut is one variety of a chronic food baby.

BEER GUTS, ALCOHOL AND FOOD BABIES

Beer has a longstanding reputation for being the cause of protruded abdominals. There could be a correlation between beer guts and food intolerance—beer contains gluten-rich hops. From personal observation, I've seen beer guts on whisky drinkers which suggests some 'beer guts' are the consequence of an inflammatory response to the alcohol itself. Alcohol also creates a drop in blood sugar which predictably leads to the munchies—and munchy foods often include ingredients from the Top Eight list.

chapter one

SELF-REFLECTIVE JOURNAL

———

• List the different diets or weight loss methods you've tried, your results and how you felt throughout the process. Why were you or weren't you successful?

• What about The Food Baby Detox is exciting, gives you hope or makes the most sense to you?

• What about your body image and health are you happiest with?

• What is your biggest frustration or challenge regarding your body image and health?

• What is the biggest obstacle in your life holding you back from your body and health goals?

• How will your life be better when you meet your goals?

• What does success mean to you? How will you feel when you are successful?

LOSE YOUR FOOD BABY AND YOUR FAT

———

We've already established that food intolerance causes symptoms of ill health like headaches, fatigue, skin problems, low sex drive and digestive problems such as food babies, gas, constipation and/or diarrhea.

Did you know that having a misshapen, overweight body is also a symptom?

Unlike other symptoms, being overweight is a psychologically pesky symptom because for many of us it carries meaning beyond physical appearance. Have you ever judged someone or yourself for being overweight? Now consider, does anyone get called lazy or undisciplined for having chronic sinusitis, arthritis or migraines? Nope. But if your symptoms of off-health manifest as fat, you're likely to be struggling with the stigma of BEING fat versus having fat. Think about other symptoms, like a headache. You don't say, "I am a headache." You say, "I have a headache." Try not to create an identity from having fat, instead just recognize it for what it is, a symptom. Because having fat does not make you bad, wrong, weak or unworthy as a person. That's the fallacy of fat.

The reason we get caught up in these faulty judgments is because the wrong foods for our bodies induce cravings and disrupts our bodies ability to detect satiety and fullness. The wrong foods also make us feel tired and unmotivated. When we feel a lack of control over our bodies and actions, we think, "what's wrong with me?" On a deep level, we know there IS something wrong. Let me assure you—it's not you.

Making a change in your life always requires being clear about what you want and why. Improving your health, mind and body is no different. Often there is a lack of clarity about what a healthy body looks like. Obviously, there are so many body types that there's no single answer. But there are some general characteristics that represent healthy.

Many people focus on losing pounds and decreasing their overall size. This mindset often results in a never satisfied body image. The reason is because there is a lack of clarity. Your body mass has no bearing on your body shape and achieving a healthy shape is more likely what you're after.

If you're intent on decreasing your size, you're likely going to fall into patterns of meal skipping, calorie restriction and portion control. All of which can decrease your body mass in the short run but simultaneously trash your shape, as well as your metabolic rate. Some people call this skinny-fat. Skinny-fat is typically a very flat shape because there is very little muscle mass present. Muscle mass and tone creates the shape of your body. Beyond the aesthetic value, muscle mass is healthy, both metabolically and orthopedically. It's well known that muscle is very dense making the number on the scale higher. But who cares about the scale? Because the presence of muscle amps up your resting metabolic rate and protects you against the most common non-contact injuries due to weak muscles. This is why I recommend smashing your scale and supporting your muscle mass by eating the right foods for your body and eating them often—but not constantly. Skipping meals, restricting calories and controlling your portions is stressful on the mind and the body. Stress is a recipe for fat. And crankiness.

Unless you live in a Zen-blissed bubble, it's likely that you live within your own unique mix of life stressors that also affect your biochemistry. Stress can be mental, emotional or it can come in the form of physical stress. Mental and emotional stress can play out in your head through grief, guilt, shame, making comparisons between yourself and others, negative self-talk, worry, anxiety or other upsetting thoughts and emotions. Examples of physical stress include food intolerance, imbalanced blood sugar, lack of quality sleep/rest, too much, too little or the wrong kinds of physical activity and even dehydration is a stress.

MODERN DAY STRESS AND HORMONES

Regardless of the source of stress, your body responds by releasing stress hormones. This is known as a fight or flight reaction. I call it ass kicking mode. Your body tends to think you have some ass to kick (fight) or you need to run like hell (flight) to survive. But, what your body doesn't know is your modern day version of kicking ass might be merely trying to digest a not-so-good-for-you-food, skipping a meal, trying to stay awake after a poor night's sleep, cranking out work to meet a deadline or negative self-talk. Hormonally, there's no stress response differentiation. Your body does not bust out the measuring cups to give you the exact dose of stress hormones relative to how life threatening the stress is.

As we established in Chapter 1, food intolerance creates an inflammatory response in the body. What's worse than the inflammation itself, is the biochemical domino effect that the inflammation sets off: inflammation causes a biochemistry-kink in your body's ability to gauge the amount of stress hormones it releases, causing an over-production of cortisol.

> *Cortisol is a hormone produced in the adrenal gland and is released in response to stress and low blood sugar levels. When it is chronically elevated it can cause cravings, weight gain, Leaky Gut Syndrome and decreased digestion, tank your sex drive, disrupt your sleep quality, cause fatigue, lower immune function, disrupt learning and memory, increases blood pressure and the risk for diabetes and heart disease.*

It's important to mention that cortisol is not bad. We experience a natural rise in cortisol daily during the morning hours. If all is well, it naturally declines as the day goes on. Normal levels of cortisol provide increases in cognitive function, such as mental alertness and memory. That's a good thing as you head off to work for the day.

In the event of a short-term threat, cortisol (along with the other stress hormones), are quite handy. The stress hormones juice up all the systems in your body to support you in kicking ass for survival. Some responses to stress include: increased heart rate, breathing, blood flow and getting your sweat on. Cortisol specifically increases fluid retention, blood pressure and temporarily shunts immune function, digestion, growth and sexual function. It shuts down the systems that aren't necessary for in-the-now survival. Digesting lunch, growing muscles and being horny isn't a priority when you're at gunpoint—kudos to cortisol for being a pithy prioritizer. Remember an excess of anything is problematic. Cortisol is no different.

ARE YOU READY TO KICK SOME ASS?

When your body is given the signal to kick ass (fight or flight mode), the stress hormone, cortisol, stimulates the release of blood sugar (glucose). The purpose of glucose is to fuel your muscles and prepare you to either fight or flee. Insulin, which delivers blood glucose into the muscles for fuel, quickly appears on the scene. For most of us, our modern day emergencies usually don't require physical activity. If the body doesn't use the glucose for activity, then the glucose doesn't have anywhere to go. Therefore, blood sugar levels remain high.

When insulin is chronically released without being used, it becomes like the boy who cried wolf. Your body quits responding to the false cries for insulin. As long as insulin is hanging around, your body thinks that there's plenty of available fuel and no need to get fuel from fat stores. Meanwhile, your cells are starving for glucose. This creates hunger signals and food cravings to refuel your cells. In a state of hunger and craving, you are more likely to make unhealthy choices and eat too quickly.

The ancient Chinese philosopher, Lao Tzu taught, "One who knows when enough is enough, always has enough."

The hormone Leptin is responsible for the Zen-like knowing of when enough is enough. That's right, Leptin creates feelings of fullness and satiety. Leptin is involved in the regulation of inflammation, including inflammation from food intolerance. In an inflammatory state, Leptin is prevented from entering the cells of your body. The mechanism for leptin-resistance is conceptually the same as insulin-resistance (mentioned above).

The lack of cellular Leptin sabotages the body's sense of moderation. It's not your fault that you just can't eat one. Your desire for more food is connected to real processes inside of the body. More proof of the mind and body connection, or mind-body disconnection in the case of food intolerance!

THE MUFFIN TOP

Recall, that when your fight or flight hormones stimulate the release of glucose into the blood, if you're not active (or kicking ass) the glucose goes unused. Your circulating glucose can't loiter around in the blood forever. Eventually, your body will realize that the glucose is going nowhere and it will reroute the glucose via insulin to your fat cells for storage.

Stress hormones also mobilize fat stores as an additional source of ass kicking fuel. Just like unused glucose, the fat that's not needed for fuel gets relocated. Both circulating glucose and fat commonly get stored in the midsection as deep abdominal fat—regardless of where it originally came from. The endearing term for relocated midsection fat is better known as a muffin top or spare tire.

Deep abdominal fat or visceral fat, such as in a muffin top, actually secretes pro-inflammatory agents. In other words, food intolerance creates inflammation. Inflammation creates stress. Stress creates abdominal fat, which creates more inflammation and stress. The result is that your fat works against you to make more fat!

FLUID RETENTION

Who doesn't hate feeling puffy? Water retention is deceptive because it makes you look and feel heavier than you actually are. You might look in the mirror, have a reflection-induced freak out and start dieting. But dieting could make the fluid retention worse. Caloric restriction can increase cortisol levels, which increases fluid retention. Fluid retention can also be triggered by inflammation and stress because it causes capillaries to become more permeable and allow extra water into the cells. It's common for people with food intolerance to have a chronically puffy appearance. Chronic fluid retention will mask any muscle definition that you do have and the body will appear soft, round or plush. This is commonly experienced around the eyes, face, fingers, arms and abdomen. You can reduce fluid retention by removing the Top Eight intolerant foods from your diet, reducing sodium, sugar and alcohol intake, drinking enough water for your body (see The Water Detox below) and regulating your cortisol levels by relaxing, managing your thoughts, getting enough sleep and exercising the right amount for you.

CELLULITE

You probably know cellulite as little dimply squishes of fat that live on your abs, hips, thighs and bottom. There is no known definitive cause, nor is there a non-debatable method of cellulite removal. But what is known is that cellulite exclusively occurs in fat tissue. If you've ever bought a massager or cream for this then you've figured out that dancing naked under the moon is far more effective at ridding you of this fat riddle.

The Mayo Clinic describes cellulite as the tethering of the fibrous connective cords that connect the skin to the underlying muscle, with a layer of fat in between. As the fat cells accumulate, they push up against the skin, while the long, tough cords pull down. This creates an uneven surface or dimpling. Furthermore, the Mayo Clinic reports that there are three factors that increase your odds of getting cellulite: stress, inactivity and hormonal contraceptives.

The book, *Your Hidden Food Allergies Are Making You Fat* by Roger Deutsch suggests that cellulite can be veritably improved by eliminating intolerant foods from your diet, increasing blood flow and stimulating the lymphatic system. The Food Baby Detox promotes cellulite reduction and fat loss not only through the elimination of intolerant foods, but also by addressing the other contributing factors involved in cellulite: stress (in all forms), sleep, exercise and toxicity.

TOXIC OVERLOAD IS MAKING YOU FAT

When bad bacteria overpopulate the gut, they create toxic byproducts that inflame it. If you recall, the condition of the Leaky Gut Syndrome (discussed in Chapter 1) allows food particles to leak out of the intestines. Food outside of its territory (the gut) is considered toxic. The body sends these toxins into a specific blood vessel (called portal circulation) that moves blood into the liver for detoxification. If you're eating a diet full of toxins both in the form of food intolerance and actual junk food, your detoxification system will become overloaded. In the state of overload, your body may resort to storing toxins in your fat cells.

Your body will resist burning fat if it means that the toxins stored in the fat will be mobilized when fat is burned. You must detoxify your body to safely get rid of fat, including fat with cellulite, by clearing your diet of foods that are acting like poison for your body. But detoxification doesn't have to be fancy or require a ton of supplements. Mother Nature has equipped us with our own methods for in-house detoxification: the water detox, the skin detox and the exercise detox.

THE WATER DETOX

When you accidentally come in contact with a chemical or poison the recommendation is usually to flush the contacted area with water. The same therapy works when you're body has come in contact with anything toxic including the consumption of toxic foods. Drink water! Toxins both in your food and the environment are unavoidable in today's modern world, but you can flush toxins from your body by drinking sufficient water (see my recommendations at the end of this chapter).

Dehydration, even if it's mild, creates stress on the body and can elevate cortisol levels as well as exacerbate inflammation, both of which will inhibit fat loss. It's also been suggested that chronic dehydration plays a huge role in cellulite not only via toxic buildup in the fat cells but also because the cords that connect the skin to the muscle dry up and harden. This causes the fat in between the skin and the muscle to pucker up and dimple.

Drink 1/2 Your Bodyweight in Ounces Daily

Your body is supposed to be roughly composed of 70% water. You can't use tea, coffee or sports drinks towards your water quota for the day. There is no substitute for water. These liquids will dehydrate you which means you have to drink even more water to compensate.

Water Can Help Curb Cravings

Sometimes our bodies will misinterpret thirst for hunger. If you're finding yourself wanting to munch between meals, try a glass of water before indulging. If you do want to add a little flavor or pizzaz to your water, you could add a twist of fresh squeezed lime, lemon, mint or ginger.

Drink 8 Ounces of Water 15-30 Minutes Prior to Eating

Drinking too much water during a meal dilutes the digestive enzymes in your stomach. Digestive enzymes break your food down and make it digestible. However, drinking water 15-30 minutes *prior* to a meal actually stimulates the production of digestive enzymes for greater digestive efficiency. You'll also be less likely to overeat if you hydrate prior to a meal. The more fabulous your digestion is, the less food baby bloated you will look!

What Kind of Water Should I Drink?

Let's start with what kind of water you should not drink. With most tap water supplies, you're getting a lot more than just water, including purification chemicals and waste residues/byproducts. Also be aware that drinking water from plastic containers can leach chemicals known to disrupt your hormone balance by mimicking estrogen. You want your water to hydrate, replenish and support your detox and fat loss efforts rather than increase your toxic load. Installing a water filter in your home and filling up with a glass bottle is the best way to ensure you meet your requirements for clean water.

THE SKIN DETOX

The skin is the largest organ in the body and it happens to play a role in detoxification. It expels toxins through sweat. Have you noticed that your sweat stinks to high heaven the day after going out and drinking alcohol? Funky body odor is usually the product of toxins being excreted through your sweat in combination with the bacteria on your skin. "Go sweat it out" is a common phrase used to reference this detox pathway.

In Chinese Medicine, problematic skin has been dubbed as an 'angry liver,' meaning the liver is overloaded and the body attempts to remove the toxins through less efficient pathways such as the skin. Toxins exiting the skin mix with bacteria on the skin and can clog your pores and result in blemishes, acne and other skin problems. If your gut is dysbiotic (more bad bacteria than good bacteria), then it's very likely that there is a bacterial imbalance on the skin as well. The real issue is not the skin, rather it's an overload of toxins inside of the body placing excess stress on the liver. Food intolerance creates toxic stress on the body that often manifests as skin problems and poor complexion.

It's estimated that the skin absorbs 60% or more of what it comes in contact with. Many of the products in your skincare, makeup and lotions are made up of harmful chemicals. As an example, the Environmental Working Group reported in a 2010 statement "Fragrance may include any of 3,163 different chemicals (IFRA 2010), none of which are required to be listed on labels." The Environmental Working Group reported, "an average of 14 hidden compounds per formulation, including potential hormone disruptors."

And it's common for personal care products to contain ingredients that you may be intolerant to such as derivatives of gluten, soy and corn. If you discover you are intolerant to any of these foods, you must eliminate these substances from the personal care products you use as well as your food. I recommend some of my favorite gluten-free, chemical-free skincare products in the Resources Section.

THE EXERCISE DETOX

Did you know that exercising is also a form of detoxification? It gets your blood flowing and blood carries nutrients to the tissues of the body, while waste/toxins are carried out. The lymphatic system is also stimulated by movement, which is our own in-house filtration system that transports white blood cells and removes toxins and waste throughout the body! Exercise inevitably leads to deeper breathing. Breathing acts as a detox by infusing your body with oxygen and releasing carbon dioxide.

While exercise is clearly important for maintaining a healthy and hot physique, it also has mental/emotional detox benefits. Exercise offers you a way to express yourself through your body.

• Having a bad day? Go kick box!
• Having a great day? Jump for joy.
• Feeling pensive? Cycle through it.
• Needing a healthy dose of sexy? Belly dance.
• Want to feel bad ass? Skateboard.
• Craving some calm? Get your yoga on.

DID YOU KNOW EXERCISE IS A FORM OF STRESS?

I've talked a lot about the ill-effects of stress as a contributor to unwanted body fat. But stress is necessary as a stimulus for growth, strength and evolution. Life challenges are stressful but without life experiences you would never discover your self-sufficiency and inner strength. Sun exposure is a stress—in excess you get a sunburn. Yet the right amount of sunshine allows you to reap the benefits of Vitamin D. Exercise is also a form of stress. Think about it, if you never had stress in the form of exercise and you were constantly resting, you would degenerate, become mushy and weak. The body was made to move! As with any stress, there is an optimal dose. Too much of a good thing becomes a bad thing. Too little of a good thing is also a bad thing.

You might be wondering, "How do I find the appropriate balance between exercise and rest?" Many people don't realize that while you're working out, you're actually breaking your muscles down. It's during the rest phase that muscles are rebuilt to withstand the new demands placed on your body. The appropriate amount of exercise for you depends on your ability to recover and manage the other stressors in your life, including getting the right amount of sleep, water, nutrition, down-time and play-time. Rigorous exercise may not be healthy for an over-stressed individual because it overloads an already stressed system. If you're struggling with chronic diet and lifestyle stress, working out can actually hinder your weight loss efforts by tipping you over-the-edge with stress and pushing you further out of hormonal balance.

Let's say you are over-stressed, fatigued or experiencing low levels of motivation. Working-out probably isn't the healthiest option for you. But your body still needs to move, just not as intensely. Paul Chek, author of How To Eat, Move and Be Healthy, coined the phrase 'working-in' to describe exercise that is ideal for healing an over-stressed body by encouraging your body to enter a state of rest and repair. As an athlete, I work-in on my 'off' days from training, rather than taking a no-movement rest day. Examples of working-in include: yoga, tai chi, pilates, dance, reflective walks or easy bike rides.

> *Working-in can provide healing rest and repair for the body but also the benefits extend to spiritual healing and quiet time to connect with yourself, calming an over active mind and soothing negative self-talk.*

If you're not overstressed and are fully capable of a timely recovery from intense exercise, then you need to huff, puff, sweat and get out of your comfort zone! Believe it or not, lack of movement can also produce fatigue and low levels of motivation. Working out acts like a shot of espresso, it fuels you with energy, clarity and motivation.

MUSCLES ARE WORKING EVEN WHEN YOU'RE NOT WORKING

Did you know that muscles are the most metabolically active tissue in the body at rest? What that means is the more muscle mass you have, the more calories you burn when you're doing nothing. Cardio training induces a rise in metabolism, but only while exercising. On the other hand, weight lifting and resistance training raises your metabolism during exercise, but also while you're lounging on the sofa after the workout. To get those fabulous fat burning muscles, your body has to be in rest and repair mode, not stress-mode. When you have food intolerance, your body is in a constant state of stress and inflammation.

EXERCISE ALONE WON'T GET RID OF YOUR FOOD BABY

Even the strongest abdominal muscles have a hard time sucking in the belly when it's bloated.

And let's be honest, sucking in... sucks!

When there is inflammation, the body protects itself by inhibiting the nerves from sending signals. This nerve inhibition affects all tissues associated with that particular neural circuit. This is called a somatovisceral reflex. Inflammation in the gut creates a reflexive inhibition in the lower abdominals because of their shared neural pathway. This means the lower abdominal will not receive signals from the brain to operate as it normally would. If you have inflammation from eating intolerant foods, you can exercise your abdominals religiously and you likely won't see results. The Food Baby Detox removes the Top Eight intolerant foods so your body can heal the inflammation, reconnect and regain optimal function. In my online video program, I show you exercises and explain how to rehabilitate and rewire your neuromuscular system so that your abdominals function properly and look good too!

HOW WOULD HAVING MORE ENERGY IMPROVE YOUR LIFE?

Maybe you want to lose fat but you feel tired after work so you skip the gym. Or do you wish you had the energy to take a photography class, learn to knit, join a book club, or hang with friends rather than idly plopping in front of the TV until bedtime? Food intolerance zaps your energy. And not having energy zaps your enjoyment of life. Here's why.

Food intolerance triggers inflammatory reactions indirectly involving your immune system. Your body funnels its energy and resources into supporting the immune system. In a sense, it's a food fight. Your immune system versus your food. And your immune system isn't the only aspect of your body that's working hard. Your hormonal system also gets over-worked—it gets tired too.

The stress hormones released in your body are manufactured in the adrenal gland. Your adrenal gland was not designed to be in a chronic state of stress hormone production, but it will if it has to. We just weren't designed to go-go-go or endure stress for prolonged periods of time. Eating intolerant foods places your body under stress every single day. The consequence to chronic stress and overworking the hormonal system can result in Adrenal Fatigue.

The adrenal gland not only produces stress hormones, it is also responsible for producing your sex hormones. Do you really want the maker of your sex hormones to get tired? If you had to choose between sex hormone production and stress hormone production, what would you choose? This isn't really a hypothetical. Your body does have to choose. Here's how it works: Pregnenolone is the precursor to sex hormone production and also happens to be the precursor for cortisol production. Needs trump wants. As mentioned earlier, producing stress hormones for survival is higher on the priority list than getting-it-on. Your body steals Pregnenolone to make cortisol. This process has a super creative name, Pregnenolone Steal. Not producing enough sex hormones is not good for your body shape or your libido.

STEROIDAL HORMONE
PRINCIPLE PATHWAYS

*illustrating the chronic stress response
/ pregnenolone steal*

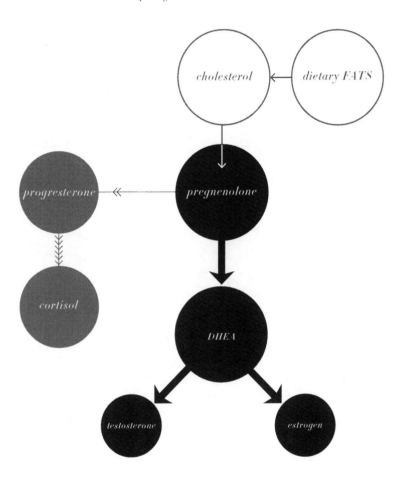

THE FOOD BABY & YOUR SEX LIFE

Babies are renowned for disturbing sex lives. The food baby is no exception.

Certainly you would agree that feeling ashamed of how you look can make you want to hide rather than share your body. In addition, sex requires physical exertion. Being too tired and having a headache are more than sexscuses, they're potential symptoms of food intolerance.

But food intolerance affects more than your self-confidence and energy to-do-it levels. It can also contribute to painful intercourse. One way this can occur is by way of the same visceral reflex that inhibits the abdominals from working. If you recall, the food baby is the result of bloating and swelling inside the gut. This connection is referred to as somatovisceral reflex. The lady parts, including the uterus and cervix also share the same nerve pathway as the gut. Somatovisceral reflex is the result of organs with the same nervous system connection experiencing the same signals and sensations. In this case, inflammation in the gut may transfer to pain in the sex organs. One study reported that pain referral in the sex organs of patients with functional GI disorders such as Irritable Bowel Syndrome occurred in 50-90% of cases. Pain or discomfort during intercourse has also been reported in cases of constipated women. The vaginal canal is parallel to the rectal canal and the compression of compacted fecal matter is a contributor to this pain.

SEVEN WAYS TO LOSE FAT

1. Eliminate Intolerant Foods From Your Diet

Experiment with The Food Baby Detox by freeing your diet of the Top Eight intolerant foods for 30 days.

Processed Foods   Sugar/Artifical Sugar   Soy   Gluten   Dairy   Eggs   Corn   Legumes

Wondering what you can eat for the duration of The Food Baby Detox? Stay tuned for Chapters 5 and 7.

2. Eat Every 4-5 Hours

Sarcasm disclaimer: Sumo wrestlers mastered the body fat fad long before muffin tops were fashionable. Sumo wrestlers trick the body into starvation mode which means storing fat for resources when food is unavailable. Regular meals means assuring your body that famine is not part of your modern life. *A good rule to follow: eat within an hour of waking up in the morning and every 4-5 hours thereafter.*

3. Sleep Your Fat Off

When you don't get your rest, your body has to keep you going somehow. It keeps you going through stress hormone release. Sleep 7-9 hours per night between the hours of 10 p.m.~ish and 6 a.m.~ish. Give or take an hour. It's not just the amount of sleep that counts. Timing your sleep with your body's normal rhythms is essential to getting normalized cortisol levels and feeling peppy.

4. Drink 1/2 Your Bodyweight in Ounces Daily

About 70 percent of your body is water. We talked about the power of water as a detoxification agent. But there's more. Even mild dehydration can increase cortisol levels, cause inflammation, fatigue and headaches. Additionally, your body may send a hunger signal when in fact you may just be thirsty. Remember, coffee, tea and juice don't count as water— water counts as water.

5. Pump Up

Muscle is working for you—when you're not working. Some women are fearful of getting 'big'. Unless you have an Amazon Woman Gene, which is uncommon, let me assure you that women with huge muscles have to put forth a conscious effort to consume large quantities of food 6 or more times a day! Women just aren't designed to build bulky muscles. While weight lifting is great, it isn't the only way to build and tone your muscles. Explore a variety of exercises until you find a way to move that feels authentic for you.

6. Be As Free As Possible from Toxic Exposure

• Smoking and Alcohol
• Plastic bottles and storage containers
• Non-stick coated pots and pans
• Microwave use
• Unfiltered tap water
• Processed foods and meats
• Preservatives, Artificial colors, Artificial stabilizers
• Nitrites (found in wine and processed meat)
• Genetically modified food
• Non biodegradable cleaning products
• Skincare and Personal Products

7. Schedule Time for a Spiritual Practice, Self-Reflection and Engaging in Activities That Bring You Happiness.

Having a flat stomach, a sexy silhouette and gorgeous skin won't bring you happiness. Exercise and nutrition are not really about having a perfect body. Rather, nutrition and exercise give you physical freedom to express yourself perfectly and contribute your passion to the world. Schedule time to explore your desires, examine your purpose, find gratitude in your life and connect with the Divine (God, The Universe or whatever higher power word resonates with you).

COMMON TOXINS FOUND IN SKIN CARE AND PERSONAL PRODUCTS

Aluminum - a heavy metal. Found in: deodorants, nasal spray, toothpaste, color additives, bleached flour, cookware .

Beryllium - a heavy metal that causes disturbance of calcium and vitamin D metabolism, magnesium depletion, lung cancer, lung infection, rickets, vital organ dysfunction. Found in: household products such as cleaners and detergents.

Formaldehyde - known to cause respiratory irritation and cancer. Found in: nail polish, baby soaps, eye lash adhesives, hair products, sunscreens. Often listed as formaldehyde, merthaldehyde, methanal, methyl aldehyde, oxomethane or oxymethylene.

Hydroquinone - a skin bleaching ingredient. Found in: skin lighteners, anti-agers, hair color, sun protection factor (SPF) products, concealer, acne treatments, astringents and lotions.

Lead - linked to adrenal problems, allergies, anemia, anorexia, anxiety. Found in: lipsticks, hair dyes, hair care, mascara, toothpaste. Often listed as lead and lead acetate.

Mercury - Known to cause damage to the brain and diminish brain function. Found in: mascaras, fabric softeners, psoriasis ointment, skin lightening creams, soft contact lens solution. Often listed as mercury, thimersol, mercuric oxide, pheny mercuric acetate and phenyl mercuric benzoate.

Parabens - estrogen like compounds are linked to breast cancer and disruption of normal hormone function. Found in: deodorants, lotions, eye shadows, shampoo, facial cleansers, body wash, moisturizer. Often listed as methylparaben, ethylparaben, propylparaben, butylparaben, isobutylparaben.

Petroleum - cancer causing, petroleum byproducts have been found in skincare products. Found in facial cleansers, moisturizers, facial treatments, eye make-up, soaps, antiperspirants, concealer, sunscreens.

Phthalates - tiny plasticizers may cause infertility, feminization of males and sperm damage. Found in: 'fragrance', nail polish, nail treatment. Often listed as phthalate, dibutyl phthalate and diethyl pthalate. These are not required on the labels if listed under fragrance.

Sodium Lauryl Sulfates - May cause changes to skin, some studies link them to cancer. Found in: toothpaste, shampoo, facial cleanser, body wash, acne treatment, exfoliants, moisturizer, hair color. Often listed as sodium lauryrl sulfate, sodium dodecyl sulfate, sulfurice acid, monodecyl ester or monododecyl ester.

*Check the ingredients of your makeup, shampoos, soaps and lotions, perfumes, antiperspirants, toothpaste, contact lens solution and detergents.

chapter two

SELF-REFLECTIVE JOURNAL

———

• Describe your current eating habits. Do you skip meals and why?

• What foods do you crave most when you skip meals?

• What are your top 3 sources of stress? Name one thing you can do to improve your level of stress.

• How do you currently feel about exercise?

• How do you want to feel when you move (exercise)? And what movement do you imagine would create that feeling?

chapter three

STOP FEEDING
THE FOOD BABY

———

Your food baby and food related symptoms are like a stray cat. You will never get rid of it if you don't stop feeding it.

The point of The Food Baby Detox is to heal your body from creating an inflammatory response to the Top Eight foods. Time heals all things. Just like any relationship-gone-bad, you may need time apart to get over it. After many moons have passed, you might bump back into your 'honey' and be totally non-reactive. Your relationship to food intolerance goes like that. Space. Time. Healing. Not always but sometimes, Voila! No reaction.

So I'm not saying to never-ever consume a Top Eight food again. That wouldn't necessarily work or be realistic. Most individuals who vow to never-ever (fill-in-the-blank) again are most certainly going to do it again. Freedom is a core human need and feeling restricted will reliably cause rebellion.

Don't make an unrealistic vow to never-ever again. No restriction, please. Feel free. Have an adventure. Do something unexpected. Experiment and shake up your predicable eating habits. Your tongue is likely stifled anyway and bored with your perfunctory go-to foods. If you feel restricted or panicky imagining life without any of the Top Eight foods, I want you to ask yourself—do those foods make you feel free? It's likely that some of the Top Eight foods are controlling you and keeping you stuck making the same unhealthy choices day in and day out. Your choices may be ruled by unhealthy cravings, low energy, embarrassment or shame about your complexion, body shape or a lack of sexual desire needed to keep your love life sparky. Become the master of your body and life on The Food Baby Detox.

For 30 days I want you to adopt an experimental mindset. That means erasing any ideas (or fears) about how you think it might go. Truly, you have no idea until you try! One of the largest blocks to eating healthy is the fear of how much it's going to suck. 'Going to' indicates that it hasn't happened yet. Fear of the future. Technically this food fear is a figment of your imagination.

For 30 days you will need to be 100% free of the Top Eight foods:

Processed Foods   Sugar/Artifical Sugar   Soy   Gluten   Dairy   Eggs   Corn   Legumes

There is no moderation—no cheat days on the 30-day portion of The Food Baby Detox. Even the tiniest bit of an intolerant food can cause an inflammatory response and sabotage the effort. You must be all in with the (temporary) experiment. 100%. Not 99%. Being fully committed is an admirable quality—keep reminding yourself of that.

1. PROCESSED FOODS

While the health of a food is subjectively determined from your body's unique reaction, some foods are just universally unhealthy. Processed foods are also referred to as fast food, convenience foods and packaged goods. But there's nothing good about packaged goods. Maybe we should call them packaged bads.

Why aren't processed foods good for you?

Processed foods have been altered from their original whole food state. This refers to the use of extreme heat, pressure, enzyme solvents or chemicals that strips the food of nutrients and trace minerals. I call processed foods bad boyfriend foods. Because just like a bad boyfriend, these food lie to you, send you mixed signals and manipulate the way you think and feel. It's true processed foods do in fact lie to your body and send mixed signals. Your body will taste something sweet and think, "Oh, nutrients are coming." But, it's a lie.

There's a little place in the brain called the hypothalamus. It is here that your brain registers the nutrient content of food. When you have received the nutrition your body needs, the hypothalamus gives you the okay to stop eating via feelings of satiety and fullness. But that doesn't happen with processed food and often the result is over-eating as your body awaits the nutrients it needs and desires.

Food is supposed to provide nutrients for cell regeneration and energy production for your day-to-day functions. But processed foods actually cost the body nutrients and energy to detox and eliminate them from your body. The toxins in these foods alter, slow and distort your cellular processes. The cumulative effect may result in symptoms of bloating, fat, fatigue, bad skin, food cravings and low sex drive. Over time symptoms can progress into actual disease.

But somehow knowing this isn't always enough to motivate a change. It's almost like we've become numb to the warnings. Perhaps it's because there is such a lapse in time between cause (eating) and effect (symptoms). Out of sight out of mind. You eat a cookie here and there. It's an occasional splurge. Everyone's entitled, right? Over time 'here and there' may become every day. But still it's only a couple of cookies. It's not like you're eating a box a day. Unless you're an addict like me, then maybe you devour the entire box in one sitting. We'll talk more about emotional eating in Chapter 7. But for now, I want you to get honest with yourself. Do you use the concept of moderation as an excuse? Are you eating for the overall health and optimal energy levels for your body?

The point here is that all of our little justifications for unhealthy treats add up to big consequences over time. Universally unhealthy foods include cane sugar, artificial sugars, high-fructose corn syrup and chemical concoctions like additives, preservatives, thickeners and colors. Let me ask you a question, what amount of poison are you okay with eating? Maybe the consequences of eating processed foods should be plastered on the packaging. Imagine big scary warning labels with pictures of food-preventable diseases such as diabetes, heart disease or obesity?

Canada adopted graphic warning labels on cigarettes in 2000 and experienced a 12-20% drop in cigarette sales between the years 2000-2009. It makes the temporary high from indulging a lot less appealing when the visual consequence is in your face.

You may think this is extreme. But is it? How much pain have these foods caused you in your life? How much more pain will they cause if you don't do something different? How much easier would life be if you didn't have to worry about covering yourself up, or hiding unnecessary pimples? What if you didn't have to fight with yourself to avoid the foods that cause you heartache (or a heart attack)? What if you truthfully craved healthy food? You might be thinking, "Yeah right, healthy food is no match for pizza, ice cream or movie popcorn!" But that's just because the bad boyfriend foods have you hooked, making you think you need them. The truth is—you don't.

The chemicals found in processed foods alter your perception of taste and make your tongue desensitized to the subtle flavors of real food. It's called transient desensitization. Think of it like your tongue getting high on junk food and numb to real food. Your tongue becomes a junkie — a junk food junkie. The great news is that this is rehab-able. Research suggests taste bud recovery takes between 45-90 days after you quit using (junk food) before taste sensitivity is restored. Once this happens you will discover flavors and joy that you did not know existed in whole foods—healthy foods can even provide you with Foodgasmic pleasure!

Everyone should aim to be free of processed foods at least 90-95% of the time. We are not designed to eat chemicals or foods devoid of nutrients. If you recall, processed foods are one of the major causes for imbalanced bacterial ratios in the gut that often creates inflammation and Leaky Gut Syndrome. Both are implicated in food intolerance.

Let me give you an idea about how chemicals sneak into your food without your knowledge. The Food and Drug Administration has a classification of food ingredients that are not required to be listed on food labels, called Generally Recognized as Safe (GRAS)—this includes the very common ingredient 'natural flavors' found in everything from granola bars to dehydrated fruit snacks.

Take a peak below at just a few of the over 200 approved ingredients on the FDA's website for 'natural flavors.'

> *Methylparaben: a chemical preservative that mimics the effect of estrogen in the body and is suspected to cause cancer.*
>
> *Sodium benzoate: a chemical preservative, when mixed with ascorbic acid (Vitamin C) is a known carcinogen.*

Neither of the above examples approved for use in 'natural flavor' are natural. And there are hundreds of examples just like this. Instead of giving you a chemistry course, here's a crash course in food ingredient skepticism: if you cannot pronounce a word on the label, don't eat it. If you aren't really sure how it's made, don't eat it. For example, you can in fact pronounce 'strawberry flavor.' But you're smart-as-a-whip enough to know that 'strawberry flavor' does not grow on vines. Strawberries grow on vines.

Be skeptical and trust your deductive reasoning to steer clear of elusive ingredients.

2. ARTIFICIAL SUGAR AND CANE SUGAR

Artificial Sweeteners

Artificial sugar substitutes were once heralded for their ability to mimic sweetness without the calories. Unfortunately, this was too good to be true. Research has revealed that artificial sugars do affect blood sugar, insulin levels and cause weight gain.

Artificial sweeteners were produced under the faulty rationale and presumption that calories are the problem with today's diets. Instead, society's nutritional dilemma stems from a lack of quality food. Consider food as information for your body—telling your body how to function and repair so you can enjoy a high quality life.

The word artificial should immediately alert your inner skeptic. Specifically speaking to your concerns, artificial sugars are known to cause fatigue, diarrhea, abdominal cramps/pain, skin problems, inflammation, altered bacterial ratios in the gut and stimulate the release of insulin. Many studies have found that receptors on the taste buds respond to the perception of sweetness with an insulin response. It doesn't matter that there's no glucose to transport, the body responds in the same manner. All of that is a set up for a food baby and extra body fat.

Artificial sweeteners are chemically manufactured molecules. In other words, they are not found in nature. They are used to provide the taste of sweetness in a calorie-free form. Examples include:

Artificial Sweetener	Branded Name	Ingredient Listing	Sweetness Compared to Table Sugar (Sucrose)
Saccharin	Sweet 'N Low, Sweet Twin and Necta Sweet	2H-1λ6,2-benzothiazol-1,1,3-trione	200-700x
Aspartame	NutraSweet, Equal and Sugar Twin brands	N-(L-α-Aspartyl)-L-phenylalanine, 1-methyl ester	200x
Acesulfame K	Sweet One, Sunett, Sweet and Safe	potassium salt of 6-methyl-1,2,3-oxathiazine-4(3H)-one 2,2-dioxide	200x
Sucralose	Splenda	dextrose, maltodextrin and sucralose	600x
Neotame	Newtame	aspartame plus 3,3-dimethylbu-tyraldehyde	7,000 - 13,000x
Advantame	(as of 2014, not yet branded)	L-phenylalanine, N-[3-(3-hydroxy-4-methoxyphenyl) propyl]-L-a-aspartyl, 2-methyl esther, monohydrate	20,000x

Artificial sugars also cause more serious side effects including toxicity to the immune system and nervous system which may result in headaches, changes in vision, neurological and neuromuscular problems, sleep problems, heart problems and many more very serious health conditions. Aspartame comprises about 75% of Food and Drug Administration adverse reaction complaints to food additives.

One study concluded that artificial sugar sweeteners are more addictive than cocaine. How can you be truly connected to yourself when you're in a constant battle with your mind to control your body? It's difficult to make healthy choices and listen to your body in the presence of a physical addiction!

Speaking of cocaine. Did you know that cocaine is an au natural product of Mother Nature? Despite its of-the-earth origins, you know nose candy isn't healthy. And you probably understand that sugar-based candy isn't healthy either. Poison ivy is natural and we don't make body lotion out of it. The takeaway is—just because a product is labeled 'natural' does not make it healthy!

Refined Sugar

Most of the last chapter was devoted to your understanding of stress and how blood sugar imbalance affects body fat and food cravings. It probably isn't shocking news that cane sugar isn't great for your health.

Refined sugar is produced from the the sugar cane plant, which is a stem with a reed-like appearance. The reeds are ground which releases pulp and sugar cane juice. The juice is then put through several steps including boiling, the addition of additives, and an evaporation process. Molasses is a byproduct of this process prior to its conversion to granulated cane sugar crystals.

Sugar intake is a major contributor and an exacerbating agent in the majority of preventable diseases including heart disease, stroke, obesity and cancer. It also plays a significant role in behavior disorders, learning disabilities and depression which exemplifies its power to alter our mental and emotional perceptions, affecting everything from learning to happiness.

The worst part about sugar is it keeps you coming back for more. Sugar addiction is a real problem. But unlike alcoholics, smokers or drug users; sugar consumption is socially acceptable. But it's not okay.

Aim to remove sugar from your diet. That doesn't mean never have anything sweet again. It means using a natural sweetener as a substitute. Many people ask me if it's healthy to substitute white sugar for an unprocessed raw turbinado sugar. Cane sugar in its natural state does in fact have a nutrient value versus white sugar which is a processed food devoid of nutrition. So yes, unprocessed raw sugar is better than white sugar. But just because it is a *healthier* choice does not make it the *healthiest* choice.

Both refined sugar and artificial sweeteners have been shown to:

• Suppress the immune system. One study found that sugar consumption suppressed immunity as soon as 30 minutes post-consumption and lasted up to 5 hours.
• Creates hormonal imbalance in men by increasing estrogen levels.
• Increases PMS symptoms
• Alters the ability to think clearly
• Decreases growth hormone production (needed for sculpting muscles)
• Disrupts the friend to frenemy bacterial ratios in your gut
• Causes Leaky Gut Syndrome
• Causes food intolerance
• Physical addiction

Cane Sugar Alternatives

Raw honey is one to one and half times sweeter than cane sugar so technically you don't need to use as much of it. Honey has the most nutrient density in its raw form. The liquid form is highly processed and devoid of its original nutrient content and is as sweet as cane sugar.

Maple syrup is boiled sap from the sugar maple tree. It has a very pronounced effect on blood sugar. Use the rule, "Just a dab will do ya" and you should be able to enjoy this sweet in moderate amounts. Make sure your maple syrup is in fact pure maple syrup and not a breakfast syrup, which might bear the name 'maple,' but really is primarily high fructose corn syrup with artificial flavors that mimic the taste of maple.

Stevia is made from the leaves of the stevia rebaudiana plant. Stevia is 200 - 300x sweeter than cane sugar and has 0 calories. Stevia based products typically isolate and use one or two of the plant's compounds that are responsible for the plant's sweetness. I recommend obtaining pure stevia rather than a processed stevia based product such as Truvia, PureVia, SweetLeaf and Rebiana. The health benefits of this sweetener are highest in its pure form.

Cinnamon may be added to enhance the natural sweetness of many foods including sweet potatoes, oats, fruit and some meats.

Fresh mint leaves can be a very subtle way to add a sweet flavor to coffee, tea, salads or even some meat dishes.

Sugar alcohols are naturally found in plants and have become popular as an alternative to sugar cane because of their low calorie properties. Many people experience food baby bloating, gas and/or diarrhea when using sugar alcohols because it is not completely absorbed by the body. Sugar alcohols are commonly used in sugar-free foods. You can identify sugar alcohols on an ingredients label because they usually end in 'ol'. Examples include: sorbitol, xylitol and maltitol.

Both xylitol and sorbitol must be eliminated for the duration of The Food Baby Detox because both are derivatives of corn which is one of the Top Eight culprit foods. Some xylitol is extracted from hardwood, which is fine for use during The Food Baby Detox. However the corn-free form of xylitol is less common and more difficult to find. If you discover that you are non-reactive to corn after 30 days then you may use xylitol periodically. For people who are not intolerant to corn or sugar alcohols, xylitol can deliver some health benefits because of its natural anti-bacterial properties.

A Word of Caution About Natural Sugars and Fruit

Naturally occurring fructose sources are found in fruits, vegetables and other natural sugars such as agave, honey, molasses, maple syrup, date sugar, coconut sugar and fruit juices. Unlike the sugars glucose and sucrose, fructose can only be metabolized in the liver. Inside the liver, it is converted to triglyceride fat and stored. When triglycerides build up they damage the liver and get released into the bloodstream where they contribute to plaque formation inside the arterial walls. Additionally, high fructose consumption encourages free radical activity. Free radicals cause premature aging, increase the risk of cancer and can trigger the onset of many diseases such as autoimmune disorders, cardiovascular and neurodegenerative diseases. Free radicals also cause inflammation in the body. Remember, a food baby is inflammation in the gut. In order to get rid of a food baby you must reduce all inflammation in the body.

This doesn't mean that fruits and vegetables are bad for you. It means excessive consumption of anything is unhealthy. To put this in perspective, consider that in the early 1900's the average American consumed about 15 grams of fructose, primarily from fruits and vegetables. Today the average American adult consumes about 55 grams of fructose per day and the average teenager consumes about 73 grams of fructose. That's over three and half times more fructose consumption!

Are You Sensitive to Sugar?

Some individuals have difficulty digesting sugar including natural sugars. This condition is referred to as a carbohydrate or sugar sensitivity. This isn't necessarily due to the food itself rather it is a response to an unhealthy environment in the gut. Certain sugars found in carbohydrates are broken down into gases by the gut bacteria and can cause significant bloating, gas, diarrhea, constipation and abdominal discomfort in sugar sensitive individuals. The key is to listen to your body!

Sweet Flavors Are Not the Enemy

Carbohydrates such as fruits, vegetables and grains should rarely be consumed alone. Everyone needs to balance their carbohydrate intake with a high quality protein and fat to maintain normal blood sugar levels. Blood sugar imbalance is the enemy. We'll talk more about how to do this in Chapter 4.

Juicing Can Make You Fat

Juicing is best used in the context of a meal supplement, cleanse, nutrition-therapy protocols, post-workout re-fuel or as a sweet treat. To give you a delineation of this concept, it takes two pounds of carrots to make three eight ounce glasses of juice for my kids and I to share. My kids and I would never be able to eat two pounds of carrots in one sitting, yet we easily drink it. The difference between juicing versus eating (or blending) a fruit or vegetable is the fiber content. Juicing separates the liquid content from the solid fiber-containing content. Fiber signals leptin-release which makes you feel satisfied, whereas fructose does not. Juice is not the most optimal choice for blood sugar balance when consumed alone. It is not meant to be a meal replacement. However, it is an excellent supplement to any diet. In a bit, I'll show you how to combine your foods for optimal blood sugar balance. Let me remind you that blood sugar balance is critical for fat loss, getting rid of food cravings, mental clarity and optimal energy!

3. SOY

Soy has been linked to many symptoms including: man boobs, low sperm count, misshapen sperm, infertility, PMS, menopausal symptoms, endometriosis, uterine fibroids, breast cancer, low sex drive, weight gain, puffiness, hair loss/hair thinning, bad skin/acne and feeling cold.

Sounds like soy is good birth control.

Seriously, soy will either make you not want sex, which is the most effective birth control, but certainly not the most fun. Or, it'll make your body malfunction. Either way, I'm steering clear of soy.

Here's why soy is linked to all of these symptoms.

Phytoestrogens

Soy mimics estrogen in the body. Research shows that an infant taking the recommended amount of soy formula is consuming a hormone load equivalent of four to five birth control pills a day! Men with high levels of estrogen have a tendency to develop moobs (man boobs) and muffin tops. There is a reason why gym-buffs aren't popping estrogen pills or drinking post workout soy. As a reminder—this is not a body image jab, this is a health communication from the body that the hormones are out of balance.

Some researchers theorize that the soy plant used its estrogenic effect as a means of self-preservation by attacking the reproductive system of anything that ate it.

Growth Inhibitors

Research shows that soy contributes to premature puberty in girls and developmental disturbance in fetuses and children. Don't waste your gym efforts trying to get buff and toned by taking muscle growth inhibitors!

Thyroid Suppressor

Symptoms of low thyroid function include: weak nails, fatigue, getting cold easily, the inability to lose weight and reduced mental clarity.

A Clot-Promoting Substance

Causes red blood cells to clump together.

Genetically Modified Organisms (GMO)

In 2010, the Center for Food Safety released a report that estimated over 90% of all soy is GMO. You might be asking, "Why's that so bad?" GMO seeds contain the same genetic makeup because they're mass produced. While there are economic benefits to mass production of seeds—it's cheaper to produce more of the same—there are severe ecological consequences including a loss in the genetic diversity of crops inherent to specific geographical locations. This happens as small farmers abandon local varieties of crops in favor of GMO seeds. These seeds increase the occurrence of new pathogen strains, pest resistance and super weed growth which increases agricultural chemical use. GMO plants may cause damage to our gut bacteria and increase the risk for food intolerance and sensitivity due to the lack of genetic variety. There are roughly 60 countries including Australia, Japan and all of the European Union that have bans and major restrictions on GMO foods.

Don't Go Running and Screaming from Soy Just Yet - Soy Can Be Beneficial If Used The Right Way

Sarcasm disclaimer:
If you suspect your man is fiddling around with another woman, soy can provide the retribution you've been seeking—turn on some jaded country-girl music, slash his tires and slip a healthy dose of soy into his post workout drink. That'll teach him!

But really, Dr. Kaayla T. Daniel reports in her book, The Whole Soy Story, that Japanese women used to retaliate against their unfaithful husbands by giving them soy. Dr. Daniel also reports that tofu was used about 2000 years ago by monks to suppress their desire for sex.

On a more serious note: Soy can be healthfully consumed (by those who are not intolerant to it) when it's fermented. Fermentation is a process where carbohydrates (sugar and starches) are metabolically converted into either an alcohol or acid. In the case of fermented foods, the resultant acid is a byproduct of good bacteria which acts as a method of food preservation by inhibiting bad bacterial growth. Fermented foods are very easy to digest because in a sense it's like pre-digested food. This is very beneficial for people who have compromised digestion. Plus it's a great source of probiotics (friendly bacteria)!

> *Fermented forms of soy include:* miso, tempeh, natto, or naturally *fermented soy sauce, tamari.*

Isn't soy a good source of protein?

It is. But it's also a good source of trypsin inhibitors. And trypsin is necessary for protein digestion and break down of amino acids. Soy's interference with enzymes and amino acids causes disruption in the part of the brain that is responsible for learning and memory. I don't think it's too out there to deduce that this is a mind-body disconnecting food.

Careful! Even if you don't intend on eating soy, it likes to hide in unsuspecting places such as health bars, protein powders, cereals, sauces and salad dressings. Read labels carefully to see if soy is a hidden ingredient. If you choose to consume soy, make sure your soy is fermented and organic.

Soy may be listed on labels as: hydrolyzed soy protein, kinnoko flour, kyodofu, miso, natto, okara, shoyu sauce, soy albumin, soy protein isolate, soya, soybeans, soy lecithin, supro, tamari, tempeh, teriyaki sauce, textured soy flour (TSF), textured soy protein (TSP), textured vegetable protein (TVP), tofu, yakidofu, yuba.

> *Soy lecithin, a common food additive, isn't considered problematic on The Food Baby Detox. It typically composes less than 1% of a processed food. It's commonly found in chocolate, even the organic dark variety. The FDA requires any food containing soy lecithin to be labelled 'contains soy.' Studies have shown that this particular additive does not contain enough of the protein found in soy to be problematic in people with minor food sensitivities. However, the jury is still out as to whether individuals with a true soy allergy will react to soy lecithin. For the purposes of The Food Baby Detox a minuscule amount of soy lecithin found in an occasional piece of dark chocolate is okay in my book.*

While the crux of The Food Baby Detox is nutritional individuality, the foods we just discussed (processed foods, refined sugar, artificial sugar and unfermented soy) are universally unhealthy and should not be part of anyone's diet, except for fermented soy.

For the sake of your inner rebel, when you resume your life after The Food Baby Detox, instead of saying never-ever have these foods again, let's just say rarely-ever. Let's define rarely-ever as being free of these foods 85% to 95% of the time.

The rest of the foods that we'll discuss in this chapter are common intolerant foods but are subject to your individual response with regard to each food.

4. GO AGAINST THE GRAIN

"The woman who walks with the crowd usually gets no farther than the crowd. But the woman who walks alone is likely to find herself in places no one has ever been." ~ Albert Einstein.

Gluten is a protein found in most grains excluding corn, rice, quinoa, gluten-free oats, buckwheat, millet and amaranth. It's possible that once upon a time gluten wasn't quite the devil it is today. One review on the history of gluten reported that wheat and other grain domestication has been in the human diet for about 10,000 years. This may sound like ancient history but according to evolutionary agriculturists this is a blink in time relative to the age of the human genome. Dr. Loren Cordain studied the evolution of diet and disease and coined the term Paleo Diet to describe a natural way of eating that mimicked our earliest ancestors. The Paleo Diet proponents agree that humans are not capable of digesting gluten containing grains. I honestly don't know whether humans were originally supposed to eat gluten or not. But I do know that today's wheat is significantly different than the wheat of our ancestors, making it an unhealthy choice for a lot of people. Anthropological data suggest that farmers began selecting wheat with higher gluten content during the development of leavened bread baking about 2000 to 5000 years ago. This is due to the fact that gluten provides more palatable textures and characteristics.

There is no doubting the evidence that celiac disease (an autoimmune reaction to gluten) and gluten intolerance are on the rise. In 2010 the Mayo Clinic reported that the increase in celiac and gluten intolerance isn't just from better diagnostics. The research compared blood samples of subjects from the 1950's with blood samples from recent years. The Mayo Clinic reported, "celiac disease is four times more common now than 60 years ago, and affects about one in 100 people." Another study estimated that for every one case of celiac disease there are six to seven cases of gluten intolerance.

Researchers debate between two possible reasons for this. Some studies suggest that the proportion of gluten content in wheat has increased over time making the gluten content of wheat much higher than it once was. Another suggestion is the rise in celiac and gluten intolerance may be the result of the development of vital gluten. Vital gluten is gluten that has been fractioned from wheat flour and is used as an additive, stabilizer and thickening agent to improve the textural characteristics of food. Characteristics such as light, fluffy, spongy and chewy. This study reported that vital gluten consumption has tripled since 1977.

> *Hidden sources of vital gluten: ice cream, gravies, sauces, seasonings, powders, condiments, sausages and lunch meats, drinks, salad dressings, health bars and even supplements.*

As mentioned earlier, grains contain Phytates which has been dubbed as an anti-nutrient due to the fact that they block nutrients from being absorbed. Gluten also contains lectins. Lectins increase blood sugar, damage the bacteria in your gut and are connected with leptin resistance, which signals satisfaction and fullness. Therefore, eating large quantities of gluten containing foods, like pasta, pizza or bread, will make you feel full and ready to pop, yet still feel hungry at the same time.

Gluten has many addictive qualities. In intolerant individuals, the gluten protein breaks down into addictive opiate-like substances similar to morphine and heroin. One unique evolutionary theory explored the possibility that gluten addiction was a motivating factor for increasing the agricultural development of grains. The theory suggests that there was no nutritional advantage to begin harvesting grains in such large quantities. The motivation to do so may have been driven by its addictive qualities and short term reward to comfort, soothe and subdue. Unlike alcohol or other drugs, people can still perform their daily tasks under the comforting influence of gluten while receiving some nutrition. Plus grains store well. Triple benefit. A theory is just a theory. But what is known is that gluten is converted into gluteomorphines in intolerant individuals and has incredible power to dissuade healthy choices.

> *Gluten-free grains: rice, quinoa, gluten-free oatmeal, buckwheat, millet and amaranth.*

Gluten-free Goodies Are Trendy - But Not Healthy

Gluten-freedom is awesome. But stuffing down gluten-free cookies, cakes, pastries, pastas and breads can cause significant weight gain.

Most people eat far too many grains to begin with so swapping your old choices to the gluten-free version may not provide you with the results you're hoping for. Many 'gluten-free' foods are made with starches (often processed) that raise blood sugar. Some of the most popular gluten-free starch substitutes include potato starch, rice flour, tapioca and cornstarch. I recommend that these foods be consumed infrequently. Don't justify your choices under the facade of gluten-freedom. Gluten or no gluten, a cupcake is still a cupcake.

Gluten-Free Substitutes

You can still eat many of your same foods or at least get the same flavors in gluten-free form. I'm from New Orleans, which sometimes feels like the land of all things gluten-laden. Most of my favorite home-town dishes involve adding flour as a thickener (a roux) or dishes served over pasta. Today my kids and I enjoy many of my family's traditional recipes served over spaghetti squash instead of pasta. Almost any recipe can substitute wheat flour for coconut flour, almond flour or arrowroot. My kids get sandwiches in their lunches except there's no bread! Okay, actually they get rollups wrapped in lettuce, rice paper or seaweed paper. 'Bread' can be made out of cauliflower which I use as the base for pizza, quiche or meat pies. This is not a recipe book, although Chapter 7 provides you with quick, easy and practical recipes to make The Food Baby Detox happen for real world people.

For those individuals who discover that they are unaffected by gluten, it is important to seek out sprouted whole grains, indicated on a label as 'sprouted.' The process of sprouting neutralizes the phytates inherent in grains and enhances digestion so you can get the nutrient benefit of the grain.

5. DAIRY

Food sensitivity to dairy products occurs when an individual is reactive to one or both of the milk proteins, casein and/or whey. Not to be confused with lactose intolerance, which is an enzyme deficiency. We'll talk about both forms of negative food responses and how healing your gut on The Food Baby Detox may heal your relationship with dairy.

Are Humans Supposed To Consume Dairy?

As mammals, our first food is milk from our mothers. Our bodies internally produce an enzyme called lactase which breaks down the milk sugar, lactose, into simple sugars, glucose and galactose. Lactose intolerance can occur when there is insufficient lactase for digestion. There are a couple of reasons for lactose intolerance: age, Leaky Gut Syndrome and genetic intolerance.

There is a normal decline in internal lactase production with age. After early childhood, internal lactase production declines significantly as milk is no longer the dominant form of nutrition. If you don't use lactase, your body halts production.

But, is it possible to continue a healthy production of lactase if you continue to drink milk?

Studies on indigenous cultures have found that people in colder climates used raw dairy as a sustainable food source during the winter months to ferment foods for storage. Cultured dairy has also been heralded across many cultures as a healing food because of its friendly bacterial properties. There isn't any evidence to suggest that lactose intolerance was an issue in these cultures.

You may be wondering why lactose intolerance is so widespread today? As we discussed earlier, the state of our gut health is severely compromised in most individuals due to food processing, stress and lack of variety in the diet. But even with an unprocessed food diet, many indigenous people eating their native diets were not able to healthfully consume dairy. This was due to a genetic intolerance.

Research has identified that some ethnicities genetically cannot digest milk after breastfeeding has ceased. This includes people of Japanese and African descent. It is worth mentioning that all people, regardless of genetics, were designed to drink their mother's milk. Babies who appear to be intolerant to their mother's milk are more likely suffering from intolerance to something in the mother's diet that is transferred through the mother's milk. Additionally, some individuals who are intolerant to cow's milk can successfully consume goat, lamb, camel or other forms of milk.

There is anthropological evidence of both successful and unsuccessful dairy consumption. This is why I don't believe in a one-size-fits-all approach to diet. It would be crazy to tell everyone not to eat dairy when the research clearly states that many people flourish on it.

Physically, I cannot deny that it does not do *my* body good. But, I don't know what milk will do for *your* body until you test your body. That's why The Food Baby Detox is an experiment to see how your body will react to different foods. But what is known, is that today's store bought milk does not deliver the same nutritional value as 'once-upon-a-time-milk', otherwise known as raw milk.

Raw dairy is composed of fat globules, milk solids and water. These components separate when raw milk is left out. Initially, the cream rises to the top but if left to sit for longer durations such as overnight, a greenish liquid rises to the top (called whey, which is used in fermenting) and the heavier milk solids sink to the bottom (the basis for sour cream). Isn't it interesting that if you leave whole milk out for two to three days you get sour cream and whey, both are not only edible but have the healthful properties of delivering beneficial bacteria. But, conventional store bought milk left out turns sour and smells gag worthy.

In the mid 1800's, Louis Pasteur was hired to study why wine spoiled. He determined it was from the bacteria, lactobacillus—responsible for both fermentation and the spoilage or souring of wine. He discovered that heating the fermented wine for a certain time period (pasteurizing) destroyed the microbes and extended the shelf life of the wine—the process is used today on milk and other beverages. Pasteur later applied the germ theory (stating that illness is caused by germs) to further validate pasteurization's value as protection against food borne illness. The first U.S. pasteurization law was in effect by the early 1900's. The germ theory pioneered today's modern medicine and is responsible for decreasing the occurrence of common infections. Pasteur's protégé, Claude Bernard had an additional theory—while he agreed that illness was caused by germs, he also believed in order for pathogens to thrive they need a hospitable environment. Bernard's theory is shared by today's holistic health model that believes a healthy gut is essential to an infection resistant body. Every activity does not need to commence with hand-sanitizer—although some do. The balance between modern medical advances and ancient holistic wisdom result in the best health.

Today's store bought milk is processed via pasteurization and homogenization. Both of these processes significantly contribute to today's high incidence of dairy intolerance. The draw back to pasteurization is that the enzymes needed for milk digestion, including lactase, are destroyed. The enzyme lactase contained in the milk itself is needed to break down lactose. As mentioned earlier, our own internal lactase production decreases after early childhood. Pasteurization leaves lactose hanging without a way to be digested.

As a health conscious consumer trying to lower your body fat, you might opt for low fat milk. It seems sensible that low fat milk would produce a low fat body. But that's not the case. Homogenization breaks down the milk fat molecules which carry milk proteins through digestion. This process makes the fat molecules so tiny that they escape from the gut and into the bloodstream. This is how food sensitivity is created! Additionally, homogenized milk has a higher content of lactose (milk sugar) than does raw milk. Studies have found that low-fat dairy increases insulin levels and can lead to insulin resistance.

Dairy Can Be Addictive

Like gluten, dairy has a protein that exhibits opioid-like qualities similar to morphine or heroine. This milk protein is called casein. Evolutionarily, it's been suggested that the reason for this is to enhance the bonding between mother and child. It is important to note that physically addictive foods have a masking affect on your ability to listen to what your body is saying.

Got Bad Skin?

Research suggests that the natural hormones and lactose found in dairy may be responsible for acne and other skin problems. Let me remind, your skin is a major detoxification organ. Skin problems are a symptom, your body's way of saying something is out of balance. Dairy products are common culprits.

If After 30 Days You Discover You Are Not Intolerant to Dairy...

Some people with lactose intolerance report improvement in their symptoms when drinking raw milk or minimally pasteurized milk.
If you discover that you are not intolerant to dairy, be certain that your dairy is from a high quality source, free of synthetic growth hormones and antibiotics. Additionally, when consuming animal products it's important to consider the quality of the animal's nutrition. If you are what you eat, why wouldn't you be the product of what you eat's diet? If there was a Paleo Diet for cows, it would be grass. If there was Cross Fit for cows, it would be pasture roaming. Grass-fed pasture raised animals are the gold standard as a healthy food source. Conventionally

farm raised animals are fed diets high in intolerant foods, such as corn and gluten and live in overcrowded conditions that make exercise impossible. I recommend consuming milk as close to its natural state as possible such as raw or a non-homogenized, minimally pasteurized dairy products. Even if you discover that you are not intolerant to dairy, I would still caution against over consuming dairy as some studies have found that dairy can promote insulin resistance.

> *Great dairy alternatives include:* unsweetened almond milk or coconut milk.

6. EGG

Eggs are a super nutrient dense food providing protein for repair of muscles, organs, skin, hair and the production of hormones, enzymes and antibodies. Eggs are also rich in antioxidants, iron, Vitamins A, D, E and B12.

Eggs from cage-free and organic chickens have a higher nutritive value than conventional eggs due to the superior diet and lifestyle of free-range chickens.

The Food Baby Detox advises an experimental break from egg-eating because it's a common intolerant food due to its overuse. Many breakfast-eaters usually opt for eggs and often eat them every-single-morning.

Eggs are also used/overused to thicken and bind ingredients in baked goods, health food bars, protein powders, casseroles and certain meat preparations.

If you discover that you're not intolerant to eggs, then it's a fine breakfast choice. Make sure to eat them periodically rather than habitually. Variety isn't just for the prevention of food intolerance, it also provides your body with a variety of nutrients. Remember, if your body feels 'nutritionally safe' then it will have no fear of shedding body fat.

In Chapter 6, I'll give you a nutrition plan for life after The Food Baby Detox so you can eat healthy foods (like eggs) while decreasing your risk of developing or redeveloping a food intolerance.

Redefining Breakfast Foods

If you want to lose body fat, have more energy and get rid of your food cravings, then you're going to have to eat a substantial breakfast. Your metabolism is highest in the morning to get you revved up for the day. Your goals of body fat loss cannot be achieved unless you give your metabolism a reason to stay high. So eat breakfast and give your body something to burn! If you don't give your body great nutrition at breakfast, your body will nag you for nutrition via cravings. For some people, cravings will persist all day simply from missing or getting inadequate nutrition at breakfast.

This may seem like common sense but if you don't give your body energy—you won't have energy! Despite the obvious, every time I eat I'm awed by how much energy I have just from eating on a meal schedule with the intent of keeping my blood sugar balanced. You might be wondering what a nutritious breakfast looks like. Everyone is unique in the relative amounts of protein, fats and carbohydrates they need to be healthy. But one thing is for sure, everyone needs *some* amount of protein, fat and carbohydrates at every meal. And for most (not all) people, the protein should be from an animal source, preferably meat. A breakfast bar is not breakfast. A banana is not breakfast. A muffin is not breakfast. "But Niki, I don't have time to cook breakfast!"

I hear you! I don't have time to cook breakfast either. That's why I cook breakfast in advance or eat leftover dinner for breakfast—meat and veggies. Everyone has time to reheat leftovers. Once you reset your idea of what breakfast is, breakfast becomes easy. Breakfast is breaking the eight hour fast. Break the fast with food that tells your body that it's safe to burn body fat. If you have an aversion to breakfast, then I recommend you peek at Chapter 7 for some delicious recipes that take no time!

7. CORN

Corn is a grain, not a vegetable. Yes, it is a whole food product of Mother Nature. So the occasional piece of corn on the cob or a handful of organic corn chips is generally not a problem, unless you discover your body is intolerant. The Food Baby Detox kindly asks you to free yourself of corn for 30 days to self-discover how your body and corn get along.

The potential misgivings of corn primarily stem from its overuse in processed foods. This means you are likely consuming corn without knowing it. A few hidden sources of corn that you may not have considered include:

High Fructose Corn Syrup (HFCS)

This corn based processed food is found in everything from cookies and candy to Coke. In Chapter 2, we talked about the effects of naturally occurring fructose on body fat. Well, synthetic fructose is even worse! Unlike fruit, HFCS is devoid of actual nutrient content which blocks your body's ability to become satisfied and signal you to stop eating.

Meat

Many animals are fed corn based diets in lieu of grass or pasture. Often the corn is genetically modified (GMO).

A reminder about GMO's: Most of the corn produced in the U.S. is GMO. As we discussed earlier, GMO food has been shown to create inflammation in the gut. With a little conscientiousness you should be able to avoid GMO's by purchasing organic corn and meats labeled pasture fed, grass fed or free-range.

Corn Derivatives

Like vital gluten, derivatives of corn are used to bind and increase palatability in baked goods, sauces, cereals, health bars, dehydrated fruit and even toothpaste! These corn-derived food additives are common in organic, natural, and gluten-free labelled products. Remember, corn as a binding agent is not a bad thing in and of itself—overexposure to corn is problematic in some individuals.

> *Some common corn derivatives include: xantham gum, maltodextrin, dextrin, dextrose. Sometimes these ingredients are derived from potatoes but we generally don't get that information on a food label, so it's best to avoid these while on the detox. Be aware: outside of the U.S., these ingredients are commonly derived from gluten. In the US, these ingredients use corn derivatives as a substitute for gluten and are commonly used in gluten-free foods.*

8. LEGUMES

A legume is a fruit contained inside of a pod, which is a case with a hinge. For clarity, legumes include beans, peas and lentils. Soy is a legume. We already discussed the deleterious effects of soy consumption. But unlike soy, other beans, lentils and peas may turn out to be fine for you to consume. Then again, you may find legumes act like a musical fruit in your body. The more you eat, the more you toot, food baby bloat and have other digestive problems. Here's where nutritional individuality comes into play—everyone's body will respond differently.

All legumes, grains and nuts have anti-nutrients which block the absorption and breakdown of other nutrients. As I mentioned earlier in the soy section, fermentation neutralizes the action of these anti-nutrients, as well as a process called sprouting. Sprouting entails soaking soy and other legumes, grains and nuts in water for up to 12 hours. The sprouting process facilitates the transformation from a seed state into the beginning phase of becoming a plant. In both the sprouted and fermented states, the anti-nutrient properties are reduced and less detrimental.

You may be wondering why a plant would be made with harmful substances like anti-nutrients? Anti-nutrients are like natural pesticides, designed to make predators regret their food choice. It's Mother Nature's method of learn-by-doing. How many times do you need to touch poison ivy before you learn, 'leaves of three, let them be?' Anti-nutrients are like that.

Some of the anti-nutrients that are inherent in soy and other legumes, grains and nuts include: phytates, enzyme inhibitors and lectins.
Phytates are antioxidant compounds that can block the mineral absorption of calcium, magnesium, copper, iron and zinc. Enzyme inhibitors interfere with the effectiveness of digestive enzymes which break down (digest) your food. Lectins are proteins that bind to carbohydrates. Lectins are naturally sticky which is why they are used as binders in baking and processed foods. Their sticky quality binds to the intestinal wall creating damage and decreases the absorption of nutrients. Think of it like bubble gum stuck in your troll's hair. This leads to Leaky Gut Syndrome and encourages the growth of bad bacteria. Lectins are found in all plants but some foods like soy and other legumes, grains and nuts have particularly high levels of lectin, which is problematic in sensitive individuals. Green beans, sugar snap peas and snow peas are low in lectins. You may discover that you do well on low lectin legumes while not tolerating other legumes.

Peanuts

FYI, just because it looks like a nut, doesn't mean it is a nut. Peanuts are in fact—legumes. There is no inherent problem with peanuts or fresh ground peanut butter, unless you are unable to digest legumes. There is a high incidence of intolerance with peanuts because of its over utilization in a wide variety of products including: peanut butter, peanut oil and in the flavoring found in sauces, baked goods, cereals and energy bars, to name a few. Peanuts are often overeaten to the exclusion of the many nuts and seeds offered by Mother Nature.

> *Peanut alternatives: pistachios, cashews, almonds, pecans, walnuts, macadamia, brazil nuts, pumpkin seeds, pine nuts and sunflower seeds.*

Foods You Eat All Of The Time

As discussed throughout this book, the Top Eight culprit foods are foods that most commonly create negative responses. This doesn't mean they are the only foods that can cause a problematic response. You may want to (optionally) experiment with freeing your diet of any foods that you habitually eat—for the duration of The Food Baby Detox. For example, let's say you have a thing for apples and you've eaten them every day for the past five years. Or maybe you use garlic in everything. You may want to experimentally give yourself a 30-day break and see how your body feels.

SELF-REFLECTIVE JOURNAL

———

• What processed foods have you been consuming that you thought were healthy?

• How many of your foods contain 'natural flavors?'

• How do you feel about redefining your breakfast food choices?

• What food do you think will be the most challenging to be free from? Why? What does that food mean to you?

• Think about your day-to-day food consumption. Which foods do you consume habitually? Every. Single. Day.

chapter four

KICK YOUR CRAVINGS

———

I want you to be successful on The Food Baby Detox. That means finally self-discovering what foods work for your unique body. No more questions or confusion about what you should or shouldn't eat to get the body you want and the healthy energy you deserve.

Success goes beyond knowing what to do. And success goes beyond putting your knowledge into action.

I believe that real results and true success happen when your natural desires match your actions. I want you to think chicken and eat chicken. Think spinach and eat spinach. Not think cookies and eat chicken. I don't want you to feel conflicted—thinking about chips and dips but eating broccoli. I also don't want you to feel deprived or to go through withdrawals. My dream for you is that you find the place inside of you where health flows easily by choosing foods that support who you already are—brilliant and beautiful.

In order to match your desires for health, happiness and hotness with your actions, you will have to heal the root cause of your cravings. In this chapter we'll talk about physical cravings. In Chapter 7, we'll explore ways you can soothe the emotional needs behind food cravings. Both physical and emotional cravings are responsible for poor nutritional choices, a distaste for healthy food and lack of willpower. Kicking your cravings will free you to enjoy healthy food—and that enjoyment will make healthy choices come more easily.

The five causes for physical cravings are:
• Food intolerance
• The wrong nutrition for YOU
• Thirst
• Lack of Sleep
• Stress

Balancing your physical cravings is the first step to recovering your ability to make healthy nutritional choices without feeling forced or deprived. When your physical body feels robust and stable, it is easier to address the emotional or stress-related root of cravings. Of course, if you feel eager and ready to tackle your cravings head-on, you can address both varieties of cravings simultaneously!

FOOD RELATIONSHIPS

Most of us don't consider our relationship with food as interactive. But it is. Not every food will be compatible with every body. Think of your relationship with food in terms of astrological compatibility— some love matches are inherently easy while others will never work. If a relationship is not right for you, you will get signs and symptoms to let you know that things are not working. Have you ever been infatuated with someone? Have you noticed that the temporary euphoria of being infatuated spell-binds you to turn a blind-eye to the irritating nuances of that person. Food infatuation is the same. We rationalize the irritations as coincidental. Overtime, little symptoms that were once easy to ignore turn into a state of disease that just cannot be ignored. Headaches. Heartaches (or attacks). Pains in the ass (aka digestive problems). Plus, infatuation does not fulfill you. When you're not fulfilled or feeling full, you will always crave more or feel empty. You will feel like something is missing. Choosing compatible foods is the answer to feeling fulfilled, eliminating cravings and creating an enjoyable, satisfying relationship with your food.

I can offer you a method to self-discover your compatible foods. It starts with freeing your diet from the Top Eight foods. Remember, the Top Eight foods may disrupt your body's ability to communicate clearly with you about what it needs or doesn't need. All great relationships require clear communication—your food-body relationship is no different.

The Top Eight foods:

Processed Foods   Sugar/Artifical Sugar   Soy   Gluten   Dairy   Eggs   Corn   Legumes

FOOD INTOLERANCE + ADDICTION

Food intolerance creates an inflammatory response that signals the release of analgesic peptides (pain numbing hormones), to protect you from feeling pain. One of these pain numbing hormones are endorphins, which is very similar to morphine in structure. Most people know that morphine is very potent and also addictive. Another hormone that plays a similar analgesic role is enkephalin, which mimics marijuana. Research shows that the release of this chemical cocktail in response to eating an inflammatory food can create an addiction to the very foods that are harming you. Additionally, the majority of people with food addictions choose carbohydrates as their addiction-food. Carbohydrate consumption temporarily elevates serotonin which is a 'feel good' chemical. One study showed that food addicts typically have low serotonin levels and carbohydrates give them a temporary serotonin-boost. Carbohydrate rich foods like spaghetti, pasta, pizza, french fried potatoes, muffins, cakes and biscuits are called 'comfort foods' for a reason.

Just as your body's reaction to the Top Eight foods is individualized, your requirements for macronutrients (carbohydrates, proteins and fats) are also individualized. While everyone needs some form of all of these macronutrients; the kinds, the amounts and the ratios will vary per individual. This concept is called nutritional individuality.

YOU ARE ONE-OF-A-KIND

The crux of nutritional individuality is eating what your ancestors would have eaten. I know this sounds strikingly similar to the Paleo Diet concept. I like to think of nutritional individuality as a customized Paleo Diet. Nutritional individuality goes one step further and identifies what kind of caveman you are. After all, all cavemen were not the same.

Way back when—before travel was available, people were born, married and procreated in the same geographical location. They ate what was inherent to the land. Over time their genetics adapted for optimal survival in their environment. Consider the life of an indigenous Eskimo. They would have eaten a diet predominant in meat and fat: whale blubber, seal and fish. Maybe some sea kelp as it was available. The indigenous diet of a tribe living along the equator would have subsisted off a primarily fruit and veggie based diet (a.k.a carbohydrates). Two cavemen with very different diets! Consider, I just gave you examples of two different extremes within an unlimited sea of potential dietary needs. The research of Dr. Weston A. Price showed that indigenous tribes from across the globe rarely experienced the modern diseases that are prevalent today, when eating their native diets. Today we're all like mutts. We don't know where we came from or what kind of caveman genetics we're wired with. The good news is that you don't need to know. You only need to listen to your body.

LISTEN TO YOUR BODY

First you have to remove anything that will block your ability to interpret the subtle messages your body sends you about what it needs to be healthy, such as B.B.F's, Bad Boyfriend Foods (processed food), the Top Eight foods or any other food you've determined doesn't jive well with you. Every time you eat, your body responds physically, mentally and emotionally. If you received the right nutrition for your body then you will feel balanced and energetic in your body and mind. But if you did not receive the right nutrition for your body then you will feel imbalanced. Using the Mind-Body Language Guide below, you can identify how your meals affect your physical and mental state of being. There's a spectrum of the different levels of energy you might experience, with tired and wired representing the two extremes. This might sound obvious, but anything other than mind-body balance is an imbalance. Remember, that I'm referring to your body's response to food here. There are other reasons that a person might experience feeling imbalanced, tired or wired. Learning to listen to your body so you can nourish it for the best health possible — *for you*, is the essence of the The Food Baby Detox.

Mind-Body Language Guide {A guide to listening to your mind-body responses to food.}

Tired State of Mind-Body:
slow, space cadet, lacks focus, lethargic, sluggish, exhausted, apathetic, socially-reclusive, Debbie-Downer.

Balanced State of Mind-Body:
Fueled, energetic, radiant, dynamic, lively, spry, peppy, full of life, stable, strong, reliable, steady, clear, decisive, focused, satisfied, no cravings, no desire for more food.

Wired State of Mind-Body:
scatter-brain, monkey mind, lacks focus, jittery, nervous, hyper yet exhausted, anxious, irritable, stir-crazy, stewing, manic.

I'm sure you can remember a time when you ate a meal that left you feeling tired, lethargic and sluggish. Or perhaps you've eaten something that resulted in you feeling wired, jittery or stir-crazy? These reactions were not coincidental. This is your body telling you about what foods and in what ratios of carbohydrates, proteins and fats are good for *you*.

Not every imbalanced meal will result in an extreme version of tired or wired. Just because you're not totally wiped out or jumping out of your skin, doesn't mean you should ignore the subtle messages your body sends you. Tired or wired mind-body responses can show up in a variety of ways as referenced in the Mind-Body Language Guide above.

Maybe you haven't paid that much attention to how your body feels. Or maybe you don't remember the details. That's okay. Referencing the Mind-Body Language Guide after you eat is a simple way to reconnect and learn the art of listening to your body. Begin by asking yourself, "how do I feel?" Ask yourself first thing in the morning, before every meal and after every meal. Use the questionnaire at the end of this chapter to record your feelings along with what you ate. Record the ratio of carbohydrates to protein and fat. It won't take long before you start self-discovering your body's patterns, most compatible foods and food ratios.

INCLUDE A PROTEIN, FAT AND CARBOHYDRATE AS PART OF EVERY MEAL

The types of foods you choose are important. But it's not the whole picture. As mentioned earlier, you can eat a ton of all natural fruits, veggies and grains and have an imbalance in blood sugar levels. Although less common, eating too much protein can also imbalance blood sugar levels—but most people aren't binging on chicken or fish. Your body needs a unique balance of protein and fat relative to the amount of carbohydrates you consume. That unique balance is based off your nutritional individuality (mentioned previously). Are you an Eskimo, an equatorial tribalist or somewhere in between? Only your body can tell you.

PROTEIN

Protein insufficiency is rampant. Notice I said insufficient, not deficient. A deficiency means you're not meeting your human needs. An insufficiency means you're not eating in a way that supports your personal goals. For example, if you're working out like a beast and you're not seeing gains in strength and/or muscle tone, then you may consider a dietary-evaluation for scanty protein intake. My clinical observation is that protein deficiencies and insufficiencies are more common in females than males.

Research supports that women prefer sweets to meats. And the opposite tends to be true of men. As a trend, women consider sweets, snack-foods and chocolate as a comfort food. While men tend to perceive meat, casseroles and other hot-meals as comfort foods. The reason for this is inconclusive. Some research chalks it up to estrogen-induced carbohydrate cravings making females more likely to reach for a sweet-treat. However, I wonder how pop culture influences our food choices and food cravings?

The current socio-cultural stereotype views chowing down on a big piece of meat as a manly thing to do, while girls are encouraged to eat sugar, spice and everything nice. Cupcakes and candy have become an iconic standard for female pop culture. This is unhealthy brain programming. Repeat after me: Eating meat is sexy. Eating meat is sexy. Eating meat is sexy. Seriously, eating the right amount of meat for your body will ensure that you have the building blocks (amino acids) to develop well shaped, lean muscles.

Sweet cravings are sometimes indicative of a need for protein. It seems counter intuitive. If you need protein why wouldn't you just crave a giant juicy steak? The protein portion of your meal helps stabilize blood sugar when mixed with the right amount of carbohydrates and fat for your body. When blood sugar levels are unstable your body panics and requests a quick fuel source like simple carbohydrates.

If you are a vegan or a vegetarian for any reason—religious, spiritual or philosophical—meatless diets do work for some people because we're all unique. You can still follow The Food Baby Detox on a meatless diet to heal inflammation, implement clean eating, get a flat tummy, more energy, clear skin, decrease food cravings and rev your sex drive.

If you are meatless, be aware of the tendency towards overusing the Top Eight foods, especially gluten, soy and corn. Soy products are often used as a substitute for meat and many meatless dishes use pastas, breads and cereals as a base. If you are a meatless maven, you may find value in using a pea protein powder as a way of increasing your protein intake.

You'll know if your diet is working for you—vegan, vegetarian, carnivorous or otherwise—if you have a healthy body shape and weight, you feel energetic, have clear skin, are free of cravings, have a healthy sex drive, feel mentally clear and generally happy. Using the Mind-Body Language Guide is a great way to tune into your body for feedback.

For some people there is no nutritional substitute for animal protein in the form of meat. While it's true that protein can be obtained from other sources, such as nuts, seeds, legumes and grains, these proteins are called incomplete because they do not have all nine of the amino acids (protein building blocks) needed by our bodies to operate our metabolic processes including cell regeneration, rebuilding and building muscle. That's where complete (meat) proteins fill the gap. Meat contains all of the amino acids necessary to fuel our bodies. While incomplete proteins can be combined together to form a total tally of all nine amino acids, it's not quite the same as meat. Plus combining incomplete proteins yields more calories than acquiring your protein needs from a meat source. This is huge if you want to improve your body shape and build lean muscle! Meat consolidates the nutrition of what an animal ate such as greens in the form of vegetation from grass and pasture, along with complete-protein from the meat. Meat is a nutrient-packed superfood! This is why meat provides feelings of satiety and fullness.

You may be wondering what exactly counts as meat? Meat is anything that had a pair of eyes. For example, a chicken has eyes but an egg does not.

> *The best quality and least toxic meat sources are free-range or pasture roaming chickens and turkey, grass fed beef and buffalo, lamb, wild game including duck, venison, elk, rabbit and wild caught seafood.*

EATING FAT CAN HELP YOU GET RID OF YOUR FOOD BABY AND LOSE BODY FAT!

Good quality fats, including saturated fats, can help you nix your food baby by reducing inflammation in your gut. Coconut oil is one of my favorite saturated fats and it's one of my top choices for healing a food baby because it has natural antibiotic, antifungal and antiviral properties to help restore balance to your friend-frenemy bacterial ratios in the gut. Coconut oil has also been heralded as a weight loss food because of its ability to amp up metabolism.

A variety of healthy saturated fats are essential for a healthy hormonal system, which includes balanced hormones for PMS-free menstrual cycles, making testosterone (for men and women) to build muscle and burn fat. Yes, women also make testosterone, albeit in smaller quantities than men. As mentioned in Chapter 2, the cholesterol found in saturated fats is used to make Pregnenolone which is the precursor to all sex hormone production including DHEA, progesterone, testosterone and estrogen. Pregnenolone is also the precursor to cortisol. If cortisol levels are high for any reason (stress, poor diet, lack of sleep, etc.), then the body will actually steal Pregnenolone away from sex hormone production to make cortisol.

You can help rebalance your system and boost your metabolism by consuming adequate amounts of clean and organic saturated fats. Healthy fats also help to produce neurotransmitters including serotonin, the 'feel good' chemical. Clean and organic dietary fat supports healthy brain function. By the way, did you know that 60% of your brain is made up of fat? And healthy fat also helps curb cravings and create feelings of being satisfied, so you're less likely to gravitate towards unhealthy foods or overeat.

Now you can see why getting adequate fat in your diet is vital to getting your mind and body balanced. The next chapter includes a complete list of recommended healthy fats, as well as a list of toxic fats that create inflammation in the body.

CARBOHYDRATES

There's a lot of confusion about what carbs are. To clarify, carbs include vegetables, fruits, grains and legumes. But not all carbs were created equal. Some carbs convert into glucose much quicker than others, which puts you into fat storing mode versus fat burning mode. The glycemic index is a useful reference for determining which foods convert to glucose quickly and which foods are metabolized more slowly. If your goal is to reduce body fat, choose low glycemic index carbs most of the time. That's not to say that you need to eliminate any food that's sweet. The glycemic index is only one side of the coin. The other side of the coin looks like this: The glycemic index does not account for how much food is consumed, how that particular food reacts in each individual body or how that food reacts when consumed with other foods like protein and fat.

Glycemic Index List

High Glycemic	*Moderate Glycemic*	*Low Glycemic*
Bananas	Apples	Berries
Carrots	Apricots	Broccoli
Grapes	Beets	Cabbage
Mango	Cherries	Celery
Pineapple	Grapefruit	Cauliflower
Papaya	Kiwi	Kale
Potato	Melons	Mushrooms
Watermelon	Nectarines	Oats (whole)
	Oranges	Quinoa
	Peaches	Spinach
	Pears	Sweet Potato (boiled)
	Plums	Tomato
	Rice (brown, basmati, wild)	

When a high glycemic carb is paired with meat and fat the net effect just might equal blood sugar balance for *your* unique body. For example, a potato is a high glycemic food. But if you only eat half of a potato and balance it with a steak in the right ratios of carbs, protein and fats for your body, then it may work for *you*. The point is to create awareness as to how you consume your foods and how *your* body responds. I've had clients give up candy and substitute it with an all-you-can eat fruit diet. Yes, they're making healthier choices. Sadly, they don't usually lose weight. They eventually become discouraged, quit the fruit and go back to candy because they falsely conclude that healthy eating doesn't work.

Sweet tasting foods are not the enemy. *How* you consume sweet foods, including nature's sweets, like fruits and vegetables, will either support your goals or break them. First, be aware that if you feel excessively drawn to sweets, it may be an indication that you are protein deficient or maybe it's been too long since your last meal. At other times you may crave sweets because your body actually needs carbs. As you heal your relationship with your body and learn to listen to it (via the Mind-Body Language Guide), you will become better able to interpret the real messages that your body is sending you. It's like when you ask your friend if something is wrong and she says "nothing," but you intuitively sense that her 'nothing' doesn't *really* mean nothing.

Cravings are like your friend not saying what she really means. As you get to know your body better, you will develop a deep understanding about the real meaning behind your cravings—because you know that a body that says, "donut"—does not mean donut!

Another cause of sweet cravings is that you may have isolated yourself from experiencing other flavors and sweet has become your default flavor. Way back in Ancient Greece, Aristotle observed that the repetition of a behavior increases the likelihood that the behavior will be repeated on a future occasion. In this case, consciously step outside of your comfort zone to explore other flavors and reset your default settings to a 'listen-to-your-body mode!'

TREATS + SWEETS - TIMING IS EVERYTHING

A great metabolic time to consume the sweeter fruits and vegetables is after exercise. This is the time your muscle cells are depleted and most receptive to replenishing its carbohydrate stores. This means the sweet fuel is used straight away, instead of being converted to fat.

You could also minimize the effect of a not-so-hot food choice by planning to eat it after exercise. Or, let's say you know you're going to go out and have a glass of wine. Make certain, for example, to eat a piece of meat and a high quality fat beforehand to lessen the sugar-impact of the wine on your metabolism. However, please don't use these methods of cheating as a way of life! Don't substitute your kale for a cocktail on a consistent basis. Be honest with yourself!

WHEN SHOULD I EAT?

Eat four to five meals a day and/or every four to five hours, depending on how long your day is and how active you are. Meal timing cannot be overemphasized! Your body doesn't know the difference between food scarcity or a skipped meal. Fat storage is your body's survival back up plan. Eat full meals and eat often (but not constantly) to assure your body maintains an optimal metabolic rate and energy level. Famine is so last year!

It's so easy to work through a meal only to look up and realize you're starving! I'm not going to spin you a story and tell you that I love taking breaks to stretch and eat. I don't love doing it. But I do love how I feel afterwards. Most of the time I don't realize that my energy levels are dipping until I realize how good I feel when I finish my meal. I end up being more efficient and happier with my work. In the immortal words of Nike, "just do it." Stop. And eat.

At first, you may find that you don't feel hungry at these predetermined meal times, especially if you're the type of person to skip meals, particularly breakfast. That's because your metabolism has slowed down to conserve your energy (fat-storage mode). After a few weeks, your body will come to expect food and you will be hungry roughly every four to five hours. This is the mark of a revved metabolism.

When you've allowed yourself to go without a meal all day, you're likely to feel ravenous, lightheaded and have a sense of panic or haste about getting food in your body. Food tends to get stuffed down. In this state you don't appreciate what you're eating. With normal hunger, your body is receptive to food without feeling a sense of urgency. It feels good to take your time and appreciate the subtle sensations offered by your food. You also make better judgments about how much food is enough because you tend to eat slower, giving your body time to register the nutrients in the food you've eaten. (Note: If you can go most of the day without eating, your metabolism is close to dead! Boost it up by eating!)

THIRST, LACK OF SLEEP AND STRESS

To determine whether or not you can take your body's signal to eat or your craving at face value, you have to make sure your body's needs are taken care of. Like your friend who said 'nothing was wrong' but meant 'something was wrong,' your cravings can send you mixed messages. Thirst is sometimes the real message.

Refer to the Water Detox in Chapter 2. Stress and lack of sleep are renown for creating cravings due to its effect on stress hormone release, which send blood sugar levels into a tizzy. We don't live in a perfect world. Sometimes, getting enough sleep is not an option. Stress happens. When you find yourself in this (or any) suboptimal situation and your cravings are crazy, you might choose to use willpower. Unlike force, which focuses on denying your desires, willpower is a super power that focuses on your stick-to-it-iveness to make health-aligned choices by decoding the real message about what your body *really* needs. Sleep. Relaxation. Water. Protein. Fat. Quality Carbs.

Mind-Body Language Guide {A guide to listening to your body.}

It's important to record the foods you eat, the proportions of protein, fat and carbohydrate you ate and how you felt afterwards. I've provided you with some specific questions to guide you through a process of self-discovery. I don't expect you to do this every time you eat or forever. This is just a get-acquainted with your mind-body-food exercise. After a while you will be able to assess your body's needs on the fly.

Tired State of Mind-Body:
slow, space cadet, lacks focus, lethargic, sluggish, exhausted, apathetic, socially-reclusive, Debbie-Downer.

Balanced State of Mind-Body:
Fueled, energetic, radiant, dynamic, lively, spry, peppy, full of life, stable, strong, reliable, steady, clear, decisive, focused, satisfied, no cravings, no desire for more food.

Wired State of Mind-Body:
scatter-brain, monkey mind, lacks focus, jittery, nervous, hyper yet exhausted, anxious, irritable, stir-crazy, stewing, manic.

Mind-Body-Food Questionnaire

• Prior to eating: Do I feel tired, wired or balanced in my mind-body? Reference the Mind-Body Language Guide above.

• Prior to eating: Am I really hungry?
(True hunger is characterized by having a physical emptiness in the stomach.)

• Prior to eating: Am I thirsty?
(Sometimes the body sends a hunger signal when it is really thirsty! Drink a glass of water. Wait 15 minutes. Then ask yourself if you're hungry again.)

• Prior to eating, visualize how you imagine the meal may affect your body. Ask yourself the following questions while envisioning your

body's response:
- Will this food make me feel more or less balanced?
- Will this food make me feel renewed and energized?
- Will this food make me feel full-filled and satisfied?
- Will this food help me focus and think clearly?
- Will I feel stable, solid and steady?

• After eating: Do I feel tired, wired or balanced in mind-body? Refer to the Mind-Body Language Guide.

• Do I have cravings, feel like something was missing or do I feel satisfied?

• Record what foods you ate.

• What was the general ratio of carbohydrate, protein and fat on your plate? Draw a picture of your plate.

• Experiment with different relative proportions of protein, fat and carbohydrates.

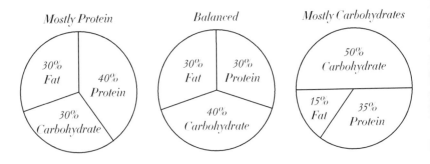

• Record how you feel after eating a meal that consists of proportionately more meat and fat than carbs. Then reverse the ratio and experiment with how you feel eating more carbs than meat and fat. Try a 50/50 split with equal proportions of meat and fat to carbs.

SELF-REFLECTIVE JOURNAL

• Do you feel like you listen to your body and validate its needs? Or do you push your body to perform when it's tired and needs rest?

• Do you blow off exercise when your body feels the need to move because you feel pressured to run errands, be with your family or other obligations?

• After experimenting with different food ratios, what kind of cave-person do you think you are? Do you feel you need more protein, fat, carbs or an even mix to achieve your personal mind-body balance?

• Describe a meal that made you feel imbalanced. What did that feel like for you?

• Describe a meal that made you feel balanced. What did that feel like for you?

chapter five

THE DETOX
GUIDELINES

———

Let The Food Baby Detox Begin!

You are now ready for the self-discovery experiment that will change your body shape, help you lose body fat, clear up your skin, get rid of your food cravings, improve your sex life and score you amazing energy! Remember, this is not a diet. It's really about learning how to listen to your unique body.

STEP 1. ELIMINATE

Experimentally be free from the Top Eight culprit-foods!

Processed Foods   Sugar/Artifical Sugar   Soy   Gluten   Dairy   Eggs   Corn   Legumes

For 30 days your diet will need to be 100% free of these culprit-foods. Let me remind, you are either in or you are out. A full commitment for 30 days is required. Moderation will not work. Moderately consuming the Top Eight culprit foods will only spark up an inflammatory response.

If you accidentally get a nibble of a Top Eight food, continue on anyway. Don't give up. You might have caught the contradiction in my instructions above. Don't waiver from the plan but if you do—keep going. The reason is because at the end of the 30-day healing phase, you will reintroduce the Top Eight foods to see if you are still reactive. Your chances of being reactive are obviously higher if you've eaten outside of the parameters for The Food Baby Detox.

One of my biggest intentions for this detox is to help you learn to listen to your body so you can determine your own nutritional and health needs. Food intolerance disconnects your ability to listen to your body, another reason why I want you to be 100% committed for the entire duration of the detox. If you are still reactive to a particular food, you will likely need to eliminate that food for another 30 days. Then experimentally reintroduce the food. Still reactive? Eliminate it for another 30 days.

The elimination period will vary depending on how long you've been eating the particular intolerant food and the amount of damage that's present inside of your gut wall. For some people a 30-day elimination is sufficient. Others may need 90 days, six months and in some cases a full year. There is also the possibility of a genetic intolerance. Genetic intolerance means that your body is simply not capable of tolerating a particular food—ever. Having said that, I'm genetically intolerant to gluten and have noticed that if every aspect of my health is spot-on, I can recover fairly quickly (within a week) from having something gluten-esque once in a while. I define once-in-a-while as once every four to six months or no more than three times per year. Just because I recover quickly does not mean that eating an intolerant food is healthy for me. These foods will still give me food baby bloating and extreme fatigue. Luckily for me, feeling bad is enough impetus to say no and not feel like I'm missing out. This is my body. Your body may be more or less sensitive. The take-away here is that once you're post 30 days on The Food Baby Detox, I don't want you to make excuses to eat in a way that's not healthy for your body. I also don't want you to think that if you eat a piece of your best friend's wedding cake you'll be ruined.

My personal preference is to pass on special occasion food because I believe that special occasions require me to be at my best so I can be fully engaged in the celebration. I feel that eating food that makes me feel bad is not celebrating anything. That might not be your preference. And that's okay. Just be honest with yourself about what your body is really saying to you and what you truly want. Not what you temporarily desire. Always remember, eating a certain way doesn't define who you are but it certainly plays a supportive role in creating the best version of you. Eating is your fuel so you can live your life with optimal health, energy and positivity. From this mindset, healthy-for-you choices will come a lot easier.

There will be no re-introduction to sugar, artificial sugar or processed foods. I do not recommend these foods whatsoever. We already know that these foods are not healthy for anyone. These foods are also largely responsible for damaging the friendly bacteria in the gut. The difference between the The Food Baby Detox and other detoxes is that this detox is about cleaning your body so you can listen to your body and feed it for life. You don't want your fantastic results to have an expiration date. You want to have freedom from not having to worry about food, health or body image issues.

What The Health Am I Supposed To Eat?

Whenever I would get into a food rut and start serving up the same meals, my former husband would jokingly say, "I wish God would make some different animals to eat." Okay, while this comment was very sarcastic, he had a point. There are literally hundreds of foods to choose from. Yet we get stuck in food ruts. Food ruts don't have to happen. Variety is one of the most critical components of The Food Baby Detox.

STEP 2. ROTATE YOUR FOODS

If your diet has been primarily composed of the same foods this is your opportunity to break free of your food rut. Recall that a large contributor to food sensitivity is lack of variety. For this reason, it's important to give your body a break from a particular food before consuming it again. It typically takes 36-48 hours before a food makes its rounds through the body, from beginning to end. People with slower bowel function will take up to 72 hours or more before completely eliminating the food from their bodies.

That's why I recommend waiting four days after consuming a food before consuming it again. This is called a rotation diet because you rotate through the foods you consume. This doesn't mean you can only eat a particular food one time in four days. It means you only eat a food for one day or up to six consecutive meals before switching to different foods. While on a rotation diet your immune system gets a staycation—a break from work while staying in town and available if needed.

I know this may be sounding like one more thing to add to your already busy life. But food rotation is not complicated. Actually it's quite practical, intuitive and it saves time once you understand it. In this chapter, I'll guide you through a very easy process to create yummy variety in your diet while creating an efficient weekly menu (in less than five minutes) that also doubles as your grocery list.

In Chapter 7, I'll share my super easy in-the-kitchen habits, meal-strategies and some recipe suggestions for minimalist chefs.

Rotation diets involve rotating foods that share similar protein structures and therefore, are digested in a similar manner. The grouping of these similarly structured foods are called taxonomy families. For extremely sensitive people who are intolerant to many foods a strict rotation diet is essential. However, for most people this is not a necessary or even a practical approach as it requires too much thought and preparation. I've observed with my clients that even if a health practice is ideal, if it's not practical, it will never get put into action. And results can only happen with action. I want to see you in action getting results! So I've created a simple four day food rotation that anyone can follow without much thought at all. The intention of my version of a rotation diet is to get a variety of nutrients in the diet, give the body a healing break and prevent the development of future food sensitivities.

I've broken down your protein choices into categories, called families, shown below. For example, you'll notice that chicken, duck, pheasant, quail, cornish game hen and turkey are grouped into one family. The red meat family is composed of beef, buffalo, goat and lamb. Fish is pretty open ended. Pork stands alone. If you don't eat pork, you could eat wild game including duck, goose, rabbit, alligator or venison—all of which you can order online from small farms. If you eat from one family on Monday you would not eat from the same family again until the next cycle begins, Day 5, or as shown below.

Monday or Day 1	*Tuesday or Day 2*	*Wednesday or Day 3*	*Thursday or Day 4*	*Friday or Day 5*
Fowl Family	Red Meat Family	Fish/Seafood Family	Pork Family	Wild Game Family or start over with Fowl
Chicken Turkey Pheasant Quail Cornish Game Hen	Beef Buffalo Goat Lamb	Fish Shrimp Shellfish	Pork	Wild Game if available Fowl

Although it's ideal to rotate all foods according to taxonomy families, I have not included the carbohydrate taxonomy families as something I recommend as a do-it-yourself-method. The reason is that it requires significantly more thought because there are more options to choose from. Additionally, I've found that for most people it's sufficient just to generally not eat the same food except once every four days. I recommend rotating the families of meat, nuts and seeds and commonly used starches because there are fewer options, which increases the likelihood of over consuming a particular food. A strict rotation diet would also separate carbohydrates into taxonomical families, which I have included below for your fun-fact pleasure. Categorizing carbohydrates significantly complicates meal planning because there are so many options and the foods grouped inside of a family are not obviously related. For example, apples and almonds are in the same family. Or how about this unlikely relation: chamomile, lettuce, stevia and sunflower seeds.

Taxonomy Family of Carbohydrates (Note: this is not recommended on The Food Baby Detox.)

* *amaranth, beet, green spinach, quinoa, swiss chard*
* *artichoke, chamomile, chicory, dandelion, lettuce (iceburg, romaine, red leaf), stevia, sunflower seeds, Echinacea*
* *anise, carrot, celery, coriander, cumin, dill, fennel, parsley*
ginger, cardamom, arrowroot (recommended for gluten-free baking), turmeric
* *cucumbers, melon, cantaloupe, honeydew melon, watermelon, squash, zucchini, pumpkin*
* *blueberry, cranberry, huckleberry*
* *cinnamon, avocado*
* *beans, lentils, peas, carob, guar gum, soybeans*
* *onion, garlic, chives, leeks, shallots, scallions, green onion, asparagus, aloe vera*
* *basil, marjoram, menthol, oregano, peppermint, rosemary, sage,*
* *spearmint, thyme, lemon balm*
* *sweet potato*
* *broccoli, brussels sprouts, cabbage, cauliflower, collard greens, horseradish, kale, mustard greens, radish, turnip, watercress*
* *allspice, clove, guava, pimento*
* *grapefruit, kumquat, lemon, lime, mandarin, oranges, satsuma, tangerine, tangelo*
* *cashew, mango, pistachio*
* *pecans, walnuts*
* *apple, pea, blackberry, boysenberry, red raspberry, strawberry, rose hips, apricot, cherry, peach, plum, almond, cherry, peach nectarine, plum, prune*

This kind of complication can be a deal-breaker and it's not even necessary for most people. I don't want to overwhelm you and I do want this to be easy.

The big takeaway is: Don't eat the same foods, herbs, spices or teas everyday!

If you generally nail the 'food variety' concept you'll likely be fine. I'm offering you a food bubble perspective from these food taxonomies. They are food bubbles. But I know we don't live in a bubble. In this book I'm going to give you two approaches to food rotation that you can choose from. The method you choose will be dependent on how you're wired. Left-brained individuals thrive when they have specific black and white rules to follow. While right-brained individuals tend to feel restricted when boxed in with rigid approaches. That's why I'm offering you the classic textbook version as well as the free-people version to food rotation.

The Right Brain Approach to Food Rotation

If all of this seems too regimented and you are more of a right-brained free-spirit, you may enjoy using a more intuitive approach to food rotation. Be sure your food choices reflect the full spectrum of Mother Nature's color palette. You may discover that you are drawn to certain foods and colors. Go with your natural inclination for what foods your body needs. You'll know if you're getting the right nutrition for you by keeping tabs on how you feel in the Mind-Body Language Guide. Again the real message is don't eat the same foods day in and day out!

The Left Brain Approach to Food Rotation

Below is a food list to give you some ideas and encourage variety. It's not an inclusive list. You can choose whatever foods you desire out of these categories. Each food should not be eaten for more than one day or for six consecutive meals. For example, if I eat five meals per day, I might eat leftover dinner for the following day at breakfast and start the new cycle (of six consecutive meals) on my second meal for the day. After one day or six consecutive meals, you should not eat that food again for about four days.

Fats can be eaten without rotation. First, a note about butter: During The Food Baby Detox you will need to eliminate dairy, which includes butter. However, clarified butter, known as ghee is fine. Ghee is made by bringing butter to a boil and leaving it to simmer until the milk solids are separated from the fat. The milk solids are the part of the butter that contains lactose and casein. Ghee is considered safe for those with dairy intolerance. You can also buy ghee from your local health food grocer—it's typically in the baked good section. If after 30-days you determine that you are not intolerant to dairy, then you are free to add full fat, organic butter back to your diet.

Food Baby Detox Fats:
animal fat and lard (organic, grass-fed, free-range, pasture-fed)
nuts and seeds (reminder: peanuts are not nuts!)
avocado
olives
clarified butter (called ghee)
extra virgin, cold-pressed olive oil
coconut butter and coconut oil
chiai seeds

Make sure you only buy oils that are cold pressed, raw and unrefined.
Caution: Toxic fats include: trans fats, hydrogenated oils, fat from grain fed meat, canola, corn, vegetable, soybean, peanut oil, cottonseed, safflower and sunflower oils.

Food Baby Detox Protein:
Ideally all protein should be wild, organic, free-range, grass-fed or pasture-roaming.
beef, beef liver, buffalo, goat, lamb
chicken, pheasant, quail, cornish hen, turkey
organic pork
duck, goose
venison
wild caught fish or seafood
elk and rabbit

Nuts & Seeds:
almonds cashews and/or pistachios
pecans and/or walnuts
brazil nuts
hazelnuts
macadamia
pine nuts
pumpkin seeds
sesame seeds
sunflower seeds

Vegetable Carbohydrates: (This is not an inclusive list, rather a sample menu.)
artichoke
asparagus
beets
broccoli
brussels sprouts
cabbage
carrots
cauliflower
celery
chard
collard greens
cucumbers
eggplant
endive
garlic
green beans
kale
leeks
lettuce (all varieties)
mushrooms
onions
peppers
radishes
snap peas
spinach
tomato
zucchini

Fruit Carbohydrates: (This is not an inclusive list, rather a sample menu.)
apples
apricots
berries
cantaloupe
cucumber
cherries
grapefruit
kiwi
lemon
lime
okra
orange
peach
pear
plum

Nightshade Vegetables
This food family (called Solanaceae) can produce a negative response in people with arthritis, autoimmune problems and inflammation. These foods aren't bad. However, some individuals may discover they are less symptomatic and more energetic without this food family.
bell peppers, sweet peppers (all varieties)
eggplant
gogi berries
hot peppers (chili, jalapenos, habaneros, red pepper, cayenne)
paprika
potato
tobacco

Select one family of foods per day. Or if you're using the right-brain approach to food rotation just make sure you generally aren't eating the same foods every day. Aim for a 4-day rotation. Write each food into the day you plan to eat it. It's a simple way to make your grocery list and remind you of all the variety that exists on planet earth. Preventing food ruts not only prevents food intolerance but it also prevents culinary boredom and reduces cravings.

As an example if you consumed chicken or turkey as your meat source on Day 1 then you would not consume it again until roughly Day 5.

Meal Planning + Grocery Guide (Aim to not repeat a food more than once every 4 days)

Category	Day 1	Day 2	Day 3	Day 4	Day 5
Protein	Chicken, Turkey	Beef, Buffalo	Fish, Seafood	Pork, Venison, Duck	√Chicken, Turkey Family
Nuts/ Seeds	Almonds	Cashews/ Pistachios	Pecans/ Walnuts	Sunflower Seeds	√Almonds
Vegetable	Cabbage, Carrots, Broccoli	Spaghetti Squash, Spinach, Cauliflower	Asparagus, Artichoke	Brussels Sprouts	√Cabbage, Carrots, Broccoli
Starchy Carbo-hydrate	Quinoa	Potatoes	Oats, Rice	Sweet Potatoes	√Quinoa
Fruit	Apples	Blueberries	Cucumber	Okra	√Apples
Herbs, Spices	Paprika, Garlic	Cayenne Pepper, Chicory	Lemon, Black Pepper	Cinnamon, Cardamon	√Paprika, Garlic
Tea	Dandelion Root	Ginger Root	Green Tea	Mint	√Dandelion Root

Start the rotation over again—if you fancy. Of course you are free to eat something that was not previously on your menu.

* Sea Salt, fats and oils do not need to be rotated.

How Much Should I Eat?

Now you have your grocery list for the week! You don't have to open the fridge and ponder *what* you should eat. And I don't want you to wonder *how much* you should eat either. Your body is the ultimate expert on this. You should feel satisfied. You should not feel like something was missing or have cravings. You shouldn't feel empty or have hunger. Nor should you feel overly stuffed or full. If you have become accustomed to eating to the point of feeling stuffed, you will have to retrain your body and give it a new set point. Sometimes ending a meal with a small cup of hot tea can help create a ritual that signifies the end of a meal, instead of dessert. This is a nice calorie-free way to retrain your body to stop after you've physically had enough food to eat.

It's also worth noting that you should be aware of how your body responds to any food that you eat, even healthy foods like meat, vegetables and fruits. Gaining awareness and connecting with your body is a necessary skill for health and happiness. Make a list of the foods you have eaten habitually and be particularly attentive to how your body feels after eating these foods—you may even choose to eliminate them during this healing process. Use the Food Reintroduction Symptom Tracker form at the end of the chapter to help you gauge what your body is saying to you about these foods.

Fill in the top 3-5 foods that you routinely eat:

1. _____
2. _____
3. _____
4. _____
5. _____

STEP 3. FOOD-EXPERIMENT
(Reintroduce the Top Eight foods)

After 30-days of being free from the Top Eight foods, you can reintroduce one Top Eight food at a time to determine whether you have a negative food response. Remember, sugar and artificial sugar are not healthy and will not be reintroduced.

Experimentally reintroduce—one at a time:

Soy Gluten Dairy Eggs Corn Legumes

I know the suspense has probably got you on edge! Are cappuccinos and omelets back on the A-list? Is pizza night making a comeback? PB&J sandwich, anyone? Before you go setting your celebration table, I want you to have an honest talk with yourself.

I want you to consider how far your body has come in the past 30 days. Consider how proud you feel for committing to create a happier, healthier and hotter you. I know you don't want to erase all of your great results with this reintroduction phase. You must maintain a healthy mindset to continue improving. This is not the end of The Food Baby Detox. This is a way of life.

Was your goal to only look great for a month? Or did you set out to end your struggles with food, body image and health for the long haul? Don't you want to live everyday looking and feeling great? I know you do. So, you're going to have to stop telling yourself that The Food Baby Detox is over. It is not over. It's just beginning. Once you reintroduce the Top Eight foods, you will begin to know how to feed your body. Finally, you'll begin to discover the answers about why you've struggled for so long with having a food baby, excess weight, low energy, bad skin, low sex drive and feeling down-and-out about it all!

This is what my clients have said about The Food Baby Detox:
• I feel so sexy with my new body shape!
• Life is so much fun with energy!
• I feel confident to speak up and share my ideas now that I have clear skin!
• It's a lot easier to eat healthy when you're not being nagged with cravings!
• My relationship with my husband feels like it did when we were dating! I feel sexy and attractive!
• I finally feel happy in my body. And that happiness is affecting not just my attitude towards my body, but also my attitude towards life!

The Guidelines For Your Food Experiment

In order to discover what foods your body can tolerate, you'll have to experiment by eating potentially hazardous foods for your body. There is no way of knowing if a food is bad for you until you experience the ill effects of that food. Essentially, you are looking for trouble—so you know how to avoid it in the future. At this point in The Food Baby Detox your body is very clean from being free of the Top Eight foods for the past 30 days. You're like a white shirt, any bit of dirt will show easily. Adopt a detective mindset. Curious and suspicious. You are looking for clues (symptoms) that indicate a negative response to any of the Top Eight foods. As I already mentioned, you will not reintroduce processed foods, sugar or artificial sugars. These foods are guaranteed to produce ill-effects on the body and will distort your ability to determine if you are having a negative response to a particular food. This means you should not eat any food in a processed or sugar-laden form. Reintroduction must occur using the whole-food unaltered versions of soy, wheat, dairy, corn, eggs and legumes.

Whole Foods For Reintroduction

Soy (fermented soy only)	Gluten (sprouted grains and sourdough breads)	Dairy (whole, minimally pasteurized, non-homogenized, hormone-free, antibiotic-free)	Corn (non-GMO, unprocessed)	Eggs (cage-free, pasture-raised)	Legumes
miso, tempeh, natto, or naturally fermented soy sauce tamari	sprouted grain bread, pancakes, English muffins (Be sure it's dairy, corn, soy and egg-free!)	milk, butter, cheese, cream cheese, creme fraiche, cottage cheese, greek yogurt	whole corn, unprocessed corn grits, corn tortillas, popcorn	boiled eggs, fried eggs, omelets with no milk, butter or cheese, add eggs to meat for meatloaf	soaked and cooked beans, peas, peanuts, lentils

• Record what you ate and your body's response to every meal in the *Food Reintroduction* at the end of this chapter.

This is how you will get answers and draw conclusions about which foods are harming you.

• Reintroduce one food at a time for a one to three day period.

Discontinue the food experiment as soon as you detect a reaction. Sometimes you will get a near immediate reaction, such as getting a food baby, low energy, diarrhea, mucous in the throat, runny nose, nasal congestion or headache. Other times reactions can take more time to present themselves, such as with skin breakouts, constipation, low energy, foggy headedness, nasal congestion or low sex drive. If your body reacts to a reintroduced food, you will eliminate that food for 60 additional days following the same 30-day guidelines for The Food Baby Detox.

• Cycle the reintroduction of each food with four days of detox in between food experiments.

After each reintroduction period you will wait four days to ensure the food is completely eliminated from the body before experimenting with the next food. That means if you end the experiment of one food on Monday, you will follow Step #1 Elimination, until reintroducing the next food on Friday. During this time drink extra water to assist your body in recovery from the last food experiment.

After completing The Food Baby Detox process, you will gain insight about what *you* should be eating for *your* body! Remember, the answers you receive do not dictate your diet for life. You and your body are constantly changing. I recommend playing detective by doing The Food Baby Detox any time you begin to feel the onset of symptoms such as a food baby, weight gain, low energy, skin breakouts, food cravings, low sex drive or feel emotionally imbalanced. This way you can be sure to evolve your nutrition with your body for life long health.

If you didn't like what you discover about your food-body compatibility, I urge you to read Chapter 7, which is all about how to unhook yourself from emotional dependencies on food, transforming your mindset about self-nurturing and creating a healthy relationship with food. On a personal note, learning how to meet my emotional needs without food revolutionized the way I eat and live, ultimately making me a happier person!

Food Reintroduction {Symptom-Tracker}

Not always, but sometimes, your body will give you immediate feedback about whether you are having a negative response to a food. Test your compatibility with any food by creating a quiet space of awareness to check in with your body. Ask yourself if you experience any of the following symptoms and record how long after you ate before you experienced the symptoms. Ideally fill this out within 30 minutes of completing each meal.

☐ food baby bloating / a change in abdominal circumference
☐ gas
☐ a sense of urgency to eliminate / diarrhea
☐ no bowel movement in 24 hours
☐ mucus in your throat
☐ a repeated urge to clear your throat
☐ runny nose
☐ itchy, dry or watery eyes
☐ a feeling of weakness in your body
☐ headache
☐ reduction in vision, slightly blurred vision or a glossy eyed feeling
☐ brain fog or cloudy thinking
☐ low energy or fatigue

How soon after eating did you experience the symptoms?

☐ upon smelling a particular food
☐ within an hour of eating
☐ within a day
☐ within a couple of days

There are a few foods that I get very clear signals not to eat. For example, all I have to do is smell lemon balm, found in herbal tea blends, and I get mucus in my throat. I used deductive reasoning to figure out that I was reactive to lemon balm. I had a few teas with nearly the same ingredients. Some blends I was reactive to and others were fine to drink. Lemon balm was the common denominator. If the tea contained lemon balm, I experienced mucus in my throat.

It's great when you get immediate feedback from your body. However, in many cases, food symptoms can take up to four days before symptoms appear. This is an important point to remember during the reintroduction phase because a food may not be compatible with your body yet you may not experience a negative response on the first or even second day. Sometimes your negative response to a food is dose dependent, meaning a tiny bit on one day won't bother you but large quantities on multiple days will produce symptoms. Make checking in with your body routine.

In the next chapter, we'll review ways to monitor your body's response to foods that may not be so obvious or immediate. I'll also give you my favorite supplement recommendations and foods to accelerate the healing process in your gut so you can keep your healthy momentum going.

chapter five

SELF-REFLECTIVE
JOURNAL

———

• Do you feel you would respond better with a right brained, loose interpretation of a food rotation or a left brained schedule food rotation?

• What foods do you routinely eat? How will you make a conscious effort to rotate these foods?

• How did your food experiment go? Did you discover an intolerance to any foods? How did your food intolerance make you feel?

chapter six

FOOD BABIES
AND SH*T

TRUST YOUR GUT

Often the answer as to what you should eat or shouldn't eat is in your gut. Trust it. I mean that in both a metaphorical and an actual sense. It's great to listen to your body when it speaks softly through subtle shifts in your energy levels or mental clarity. But sometimes, your body will speak loudly in ways you can't ignore—like through the appearance of a food baby or other digestive problems. Listening to your body also includes evaluating what comes out of it. Your bowel movements contain clues about your digestion and how compatible your food choices were with your body. Don't discount your own feelings and urges. Examine them. Your 'gut' instinct is packed with valuable information.

THE POWDER ROOM EXPOSÉ

I find it daunting that people are ashamed of this particular body function—everyone poops. No exceptions.

Here are three questions that I've included in my client paperwork since 2009. The majority of my clients answer yes to all three questions.

• Do you feel embarrassed, ashamed or dirty for having a bowel movement (BM) outside of your home (friend's house or public restroom)?

• Do you feel others judge you as dirty or unlovable if you have a BM in their home or in a public restroom?
• Do you 'hold it' or suppress the urge to have a BM until you are at home?

I'm not sure why people have body-function shame (although I have my theories and own experiences). But what I do know is that it's just another example of how people wage war on their bodies with unhealthy thoughts. Or what I call mind-body disconnection. You cannot hate one aspect of your body or body function and fully love your body. You cannot discount one natural desire and still honor yourself. The very nature of body-shame is disconnection and dishonor. You must embrace your entire body as part of you. And love every bit. Poop and all.

As I mentioned in Chapter 2, for some, body fat is a symptom that is associated with shame. I'd say unhealthy bowels are a close second. Unhealthy bowels are revealed in many forms. Constipation. Bloating. Food baby. Diarrhea. Excessive gas. Excessive boriborygmus, the sound of gas inside of the intestines. It's a natural human inclination to feel anxious that someone will hear, smell or see your powder room aftermath. We discussed that the appearance of a food baby (from an evolutionary-psychology perspective) signifies an unhealthy body. Foul-smelling bowel movements are also a sign of an unhealthy body.

Subconsciously, we may be wired to fear disconnection and abandonment from having stinky BM's. Survival behaviorists report that prior to medical advances, humans as well as animals isolate ill members by their smells to avoid the spread of disease. Let me remind you that this theory just sheds light on why we're biologically hard-wired to feel embarrassed about the sound, smell or sight of unhealthy BM's. This symptom (like any symptom) doesn't make you unlovable. It's simply your body (using a mega-phone) communicating to you that something needs to change.

BM 101

Information about your health, digestion and your body's food preferences can be found in the toilet. It's pretty common for people with food intolerance to have unhealthy BM's. You may notice your BM's start to shift to a healthier form while on The Food Baby Detox. Rebalancing your health is the first step in learning the art of listening to your body. Once you have achieved a healthy baseline you will be better equipped to hear your body's health-warnings. If you generally have healthy BM's and you observe something unhealthy coming out of you, then think back to what you ate that day and make a mental note. This is one way you can self-discover your body's preferences for food and/or supplements. If you don't have a healthy BM baseline, don't fret. It takes time and consistency to rebalance your body.

Rebalancing your body starts with choosing the right foods for you and can be facilitated with healing supplements (which are recommended at the end of this chapter). Unhealthy BM's can be an indication of serious medical problems. For example, if you have blood in your stool, a pain in your abdomen that doesn't go away, bloating and/or distention that does not go away or seems unrelated to what you are eating, you should consult your doctor.

Signs of a Healthy BM:
Smell: Earthy. Natural.
Color: Medium to light brown.
Shape: Snake. Log. Sausage.
Consistency: Uniform. One piece. Smooth.
Size: 1-2 inches in diameter. 12-18 inches total per day.
Frequency: Varies per individual from 1 BM/day to 3 BM's/day.
Experience: The sensation 'to go' should be notable but not urgent. No straining or pain. The stool should pass easily and without much delay.

As we discussed at length in Chapter 1, your gut is home to friendly and frenemy (bad) bacteria. Guess what? All microorganisms poop, including bacteria. Ok, it's not actually called poop. It's called metabolic waste. But nonetheless, the bacteria in your gut are pooping inside of you. The metabolic waste of the friendly bacteria is actually recycled by our bodies to increase digestion and detoxification. As the name implies, friendly bacteria are our friends! Remember, friendly bacteria can be destroyed with a high consumption of processed foods, sugar, artificial sugar and negative response foods. Supplements kick-start the healing and repair your gut to make it once-again a hospitable environment to your friendly-bacteria.

SUPPLEMENTS

The following are my favorite supplements to revive your gut and heal your food baby. But remember no supplement is a magic bullet. Supplements do just what their name implies—they supplement. What you eat should be your primary source of nutrients. Supplements aid and give you a gentle push in the direction of balancing your health. Most of the recommended food baby supplements have anti-inflammatory properties to facilitate healing the gut. The other common characteristics you'll notice in the food baby supplements is that most of them support digestion and have natural antibiotic, antifungal and antiviral properties to inhibit the presence of unhealthy microbes in the gut. Many of the supplements also have a detoxifying effect and help to balance blood sugar levels, which will aid in fat loss. Please consult your doctor before beginning a supplement program and check for drug and other supplement interactions in the book, *A-Z Guide to Drug-Herb-Vitamin Interactions* by Healthnotes.

FOOD BABY HEALING HERBAL TEAS

Teas are a great way to end a meal (instead of dessert), satisfy a craving, create a down-time ritual and empower the body with healing nutrients. Rotate your tea selection to get a variety of healing nutrients.

Make your own fresh herb tea:

I suggest grating the root or herb to release the potency of the nutrients and enzymes prior to placing it into a tea strainer. Steep it in boiling water for 5 minutes. Remove strainer and enjoy.

Here are the teas that I recommend specifically for your food baby and gut healing:

Dandelion Root

This herbal is heralded for its ability to ease bloating, improve digestion, regulate blood sugar, aid in weight loss and stimulate detoxification through the skin and liver! Dandelion root may be eaten, grated and steeped as tea, bought in pre-packaged tea bags and found in capsule form.

Ginger Root

This herb is often used as a spice. But, it can also be taken in capsules, steeped as a tea, eaten or juiced. Ginger is known for its anti-gas, anti-diarrhea, anti-inflammatory and stomach soothing properties. It also increases digestive enzyme activity. (Check with your doctor before using this herb if you are on blood-thinners.)

Pau D'Arco

The most valuable part of this plant is from the inner most bark as it contains potent anti-inflammatory, anti-bacterial, anti-fungal anti-viral and laxative properties.

Green Tea

This tea increases fat metabolism, improves blood sugar balance and improves insulin sensitivity. Green tea has also been shown to have some anti-bacterial and anti-viral properties. I recommend drinking this in the morning because it does contain caffeine.

Mint

Mint is gentle and soothing. It can improve digestion and bowel function, sooth irritable bowels and indigestion. Mint can be steeped as a tea, used in cooking, smoothies, coffee or you can chew the leaves directly.

Chamomile

This pretty little plant is most commonly used in tea to create a sense of calm. It can aid in calming nausea, gas, digestion and even menstrual cramps. Topically, it can be used to soothe itchy or inflamed skin, psoriasis and acne.

Rooibos

Also called red bush tea, this tea is notable because it is caffeine-free. Rooibos has anti-inflammatory properties, improves circulation (important for accelerating the healing process), increases the absorption of iron and relieves stomach cramps, diarrhea and indigestion. A warm tea bag can also be applied directly to the skin to soothe irritated skin such as in psoriasis, eczema and acne.

OTHER FOOD BABY HEALING SUPPLEMENTS

Garlic

Garlic can be a powerful agent in fighting against bacterial, fungal and viral infections. The benefits of garlic are found in the compound, Allicin. In order to activate Allicin, the garlic should be fresh and then crushed or chopped and consumed within an hour or two. *Consume fresh garlic liberally.*

Rosemary

Besides being an anti-inflammatory, an immune system booster and an aid in digestion, this herb is delicious on a variety of foods! Use liberally and eat it raw, dried or cooked.

Probiotics

Probiotics are friendly bacteria that are responsible for a healthy immune system and digestion. Probiotics have been shown to improve digestion, decrease inflammation, improve nasal and sinus congestion, as well as improve skin conditions like acne. Daily probiotics taken before bed are recommended while on The Food Baby Detox.

Digestive Enzymes

Digestive enzymes helps to break down and digest food. Damaged guts produce insufficient digestive enzymes for proper food digestion. Additionally, the natural production of digestive enzymes diminishes with age. Digestive enzymes are recommended daily with meals while on The Food Baby Detox.

Hydrochloric Acid (HCL)

HCL is a naturally occurring stomach acid that helps absorb nutrients, antioxidants, breaks down protein and activates enzymes, hormones and neurotransmitters. It protects the body against bacterial pathogens and aids in Leaky Gut Syndrome repair. Low HCL levels can be associated with bloating, indigestion, constipation, acne and the inability to sleep well. HCL is recommended daily, with meals, and is included in The Food Baby Detox—Digestive Enzyme supplement available at www.nikidriscoll.com/foodbabydetoxsupplements.

Slippery Elm

This herb has a gel-like quality that coats and soothes inflammation. This herb is helpful in alleviating diarrhea and other inflammatory bowel conditions. It can be found in capsule form—follow the recommended dose.

Marshmallow Root

This herb has a slimy thick consistency that acts to coat and soothe inflamed mucous membranes such as in the digestive tract. It also may be used topically for skin inflammation. It can be found in capsule form or you can steep your own tea.

L-Glutamine

This amino acid has been found to support the regeneration of the intestinal wall lining and help fuel the enterocytes (the Troll-like cells that line the small intestine). It is also critical for the uptake of amino acids and other nutrients supporting protein synthesis. This supplement is great for healing Leaky Gut Syndrome! It can be found in capsule form.

N-Acetyl Glucosamine

This is a combination of an amino acid and glucose. It is anti-inflammatory and enhances mucus production to protect the gastro-intestinal mucosal lining. It can be found in capsule form.

Aloe Vera

This plant is know for being an adaptagen, meaning it has the capacity to adapt to even the most inhospitable environments—it has the same adaptability as a healing agent inside the body. It has anti-inflammatory, antiseptic and detoxifying properties. It is often used to aid digestion, support detoxification, boost the immune system, restore good to bad bacterial balance and treat both constipation and diarrhea. It can be found in both liquid and capsule form.

Okra

This vegetable has gel-like fiber that works to coat the mucosal lining of the intestinal wall to soothe inflammation. It is helpful for both constipation and diarrhea, helps stabilize blood sugar levels and is high in antioxidants, Vitamin C, niacin and folic acid. It may be eaten in whole food form or taken in capsule form.

Cat's Claw

This rain forest herb has adaptogenic, anti-inflammatory, antimicrobial and anti-viral properties. It helps repair damaged structures in the gut and restore good to bad bacterial balance. This herb may be taken in tea or capsule form.

5-HTP

This is the precursor to the production of the neurotransmitters, serotonin and melatonin, which affect cravings, mood, mental clarity and sleep. 5-HTP has been included in therapeutic protocols to aid in the healing of cravings, food addiction, sleep disorders and depression. In order for 5-HTP to be metabolized in the body, vitamin B6 must be present.

Rhodiola Rosea

This herb is adaptogenic and helps the body 'roll with the punches' by regulating the release of excess cortisol. As mentioned in Chapter 2, high cortisol imbalances blood sugar, increases the likelihood of storing abdominal fat, tanks energy and sex drive. Rhodiola also activates lipase, an enzyme that helps digest and burn fat. But that's not all, this herb also increases your sensitivity to the neurotransmitters serotonin and melatonin—which aid in healing cravings and addictive patterns, improve mental clarity, focus, mood and the perception of pleasure—yummy food and sex anyone? This herb is included in The Food Baby Detox Cravings Calmer supplement alongside 5HTP and vitamin B6.

The Food Baby Detox Supplement Program
Creating a body that you are proud of and feel good inside of doesn't need to be hard. You don't need to spend a ton of money, purchase and pill pop all 15-20 supplements mentioned above. The Food Baby Detox Supplement Program was created to help you get healthy and heal your gut in a realistic way. Everything you need is in 4 bottles!

The Food Baby Detox Supplement Program includes the Probiotic Blend, Digestive Enzyme, GI Restore, a blend of the above mentioned healing plants, herbs and amino acids and Cravings Calmer, a synergistic blend of 5HTP, vitamin B6 and Rhodiola. The Food Baby Detox supplements are available at www.nikidriscoll.com/foodbabydetoxsupplements.

FOOD BABY HEALING FATS & OILS

Coconut Oil

This oil has antimicrobial and anti-inflammatory properties. The specific way coconut oil fatty acids are metabolized may encourage feelings of satiety and has been shown to increase fat burning—specifically around the midsection. This oil is tasty and great for frying food because of its ability to withstand high temperatures. A tablespoon of coconut oil can be added to morning smoothies or coffee. Coconut oil can also be used topically (directly on the skin) to heal acne, moisturize the skin or even used as a natural vaginal lubricant. As always make sure your oils are from an organic, raw and unrefined (virgin) source. Use liberally.

Oregano

This herb is most potent when used in essential oil form. Like many essential oils, Oregano oil has powerful antibacterial, antifungal and antiviral properties. Oregano oil is a unique essential oil because it's one of the few that are safe for ingestion. The oil may also be used topically to help with skin problems. Because of its incredible potency it should only be used short-term and it must be substantially diluted — a little bit goes a long way. For internal use, it is recommended to use four to six drops diluted in an eight ounce glass of water. For topical use, it is recommended to use four to six drops per three tablespoons of a carrier oil such as olive, almond oil or coconut oil for a salve. Follow the recommended dose and use as needed. This is not recommended for long-term use (no more than ten days).

Fish Oil

There's a lot of hype about this supplement and for good reason. Fish oil, a source omega-3 fatty acids, has anti-inflammatory properties, has been shown to improve brain function and encourages increased protein synthesis (muscle growth). This can be taken in pill form or by eating wild-caught salmon. Use liberally.

Evening Primrose Oil

This supplement is one of my favorites for reducing stretch marks and saggy skin that can occur after losing a food baby. It contains the fatty acid known as gamma-linoleic acid (GLA) that is beneficial for restoring elasticity to the skin. It's also been shown to help regulate hormones, heal acne and skin problems. Use as directed.

Rose Essential Oil

A topical stretch mark, skin-sag remedy. I recommend mixing five to fifteen drops of Rose Oil with two to three tablespoons of a carrier oil such as olive, coconut or almond oil. Massage directly into skin for five to fifteen minutes/day to improve elasticity.

Chiai Seeds

Chiai seeds come from a flowering plant in the mint family. It's valuable for balancing blood sugar (eh-hem lowering belly fat), improving digestion and is a great source of omega-3 fatty acids. These seeds are virtually tasteless so you can easily add them to anything for a health boost.

A DOSE OF DETOX

Chlorophyll

You might remember this from science class as the stuff that makes plants green. But, chlorophyll is so much more than a hue. It promotes friendly bacteria, acts as an anti-inflammatory, helps break addiction and detoxifies the liver and skin. It's even been dubbed as the internal deodorant because of its powerful cleansing properties. It is naturally found in green leafy vegetables like chard, collard, kale, spinach, alfalfa, lettuce, broccoli and sea vegetables including spirulina, chlorella and blue green algae. Eat it. It can also be found in concentrated liquid form in the supplement section of your health grocer.

chapter six

SELF-REFLECTIVE JOURNAL

———

• Do you feel embarrassed, ashamed or dirty for having a bowel movement (BM) outside of your home (friends house or public restroom)?

• Do you feel others judge you as dirty or unlovable if you have a BM in their home or in a public restroom?

• Do you 'hold it' or suppress the urge to have a BM until you are at home?

• Can you focus on your body's functions as amazing, efficient, cleansing and healthy? Whenever you have a negative thought about your body functions, think about how your body is keeping your insides clean.

•Make showing gratitude towards your body a practice. Say thank you to your body for doing the best it can with what it has to work with.

• How can you create a culture in your home that is accepting, non-polarized yet still private in regards to body function?

chapter seven

HAPPY PLATES AND PANTRIES: EATING SHOULD BE A HAPPY OCCASION!

TRUE HAPPINESS COMES FROM ALIGNING YOUR THOUGHTS WITH YOUR ACTIONS

Did your parents or teachers ever tell you to make a happy-plate? Meaning the plate is happy when all the food has been eaten. This isn't actually a happy-plate. It's an unhappy-plate because if you're not really hungry and you eat anyway, you've overridden your body's fullness meter. Or maybe you just plain don't like the taste and you force it down. You'll never be happy when you're disconnected from your own authenticity, including your authentic desire for food. When you are connected to your body, you can trust your taste buds to guide you towards nutritious-for-you foods and steer you away from harmful-for-you foods.

The happy-plate mentality discounts your body's innate wisdom in choosing foods that are right for you and instead relies on an external force to choose foods that may be wrong for you. You are the only one who knows what food is right for you.

Healthy eating honors your body's needs and true desires. I'm going to show you how to make a real 'happy-plate' by respecting your body with health-connected choices and by honoring your kitchen and pantry as a healthy-for-you-sanctuary.

IT TAKES TWO TO TANGO

Having a great relationship goes beyond choosing a compatible partner. Your relationships must be nurtured and paid attention to. Your relationship with food is no different than any other relationship in your life. I know you'd agree that it's rude to text, watch TV or space out when you're supposed to be spending time someone. So when has it become acceptable to ignore your food in this way? If you really stop to appreciate food as a miracle of nature, you will find it fascinating and awe inspiring.

Look at your food. Really examine it. Color. Texture. Shape. It's an absolute work of art! Touch it. Feel the curves and contour in your hands. Make a point to smell it and breathe it into your being. Instead of shoveling it down, try biting into it slowly. Feel your teeth sink into it. Chew it slowly and allow the flavor to seep out until it surrounds your entire mouth. Feel the texture on your tongue. Listen to the sound your food makes as you chew. Your relationship with your food can be extremely pleasurable, even foodgasmic. All you have to do is devote your attention to what you're doing. Presence is polite. Use your manners.

You won't experience real pleasure unless you are connected to your body. I'm not talking about tongue-specific pleasure. Or the pseudo pleasure of escaping reality through food. Real pleasure is a divinely inspired, full body experience. And you can have real pleasure in your relationship with food. But first you have to be connected to yourself which means you have to love and accept every aspect of your body and soul.

I don't know many people who truly enjoy having a food baby, an unhealthy shape or excess body fat. And most of us end up feeling like we hate the body part we want to change. Sure, sometimes it feels easier to say nasty things to yourself, like, "I don't deserve to wear this-or-that, because I'm too fat." Maybe you put conditions on what you're allowed to feel. "I can't be sexy until I lose weight." "I can't be seen at social functions until I get in shape." "I don't deserve to enjoy food because I'm fat." And when you do choose to indulge, do you tell yourself that you're bad or wrong for it?

The fallacy of negative self-talk is the belief that if you hate yourself enough you'll change. I'm here to tell you that it's not true. Hating yourself drains you of energy and motivation. Hating yourself disconnects you from yourself and makes you feel worthless, insignificant and unlovable. And if you think you're not worth the effort, you won't make the effort. With a self-hate mindset, you will subconsciously sabotage your own efforts with little exceptions here and there. You might even feel like you tried and failed. But the reality is that your state of mind wasn't geared up for a successful effort. Forget chastising yourself. Leave the lectures behind. You have to love yourself healthy. Stop verbally abusing yourself with negative self-talk. And stop physically abusing yourself by eating the wrong foods in the wrong amounts for your body. Take responsibility for your misaligned choices, don't dwell on them. Acknowledge how you could do better and make a plan and do it!

LOVE YOURSELF HEALTHY BY VALIDATING YOUR BODY'S NEEDS

You live in your body and no one will ever know it better than you. If you don't feel like you know your body, then you have to repair your relationship with your body ASAP! How are you going to feed something you don't know anything about? But don't worry, you actually know more about your body than you think. As a matter of fact, you were born knowing your body. You may be wondering, "if being connected to my body is innate, why did I lose touch with it?" A big reason for losing touch with your body is a lack of presence. When you are in the moment, you are feeling and sensing everything—your body and your environment. You were born 100% present in the moment. Because you didn't know any other way to be. No past or future existed yet to occupy your mind. And that's exactly how you're going to rekindle your body-relationship. You will need to practice being child-like and present. Innocent. Wide-eyed. Explorative—with a blank slate and no judgments.

A large part of presence is removing judgements about what your body is experiencing—because the judgement itself alters your perception of what is actually occurring. If you are eating cake but you're thinking, "this is bad," then you are not feeling your body—you are stuck in your head. However, if you are eating cake and you are fully engaged and aware of what your body is experiencing, then you may notice how beautiful it is—smelling, tasting and feeling it's texture. If you were eating in this fully engaged way, you would also notice after eating a moderate amount that your tummy may feel heavier, your thoughts may become foggy or you may feel jittery—all signals to stop eating.

Think about a healthy baby exploring a food for the first time. They look at it, examine it's color, shape and texture. Babies smell the food, touch it, taste it, feel it in their mouths and listen to the sound it makes as they chew. It's a blank slate exploration. Babies do not judge themselves as good or bad. They do not reward or punish themselves. They take no more pride in eating a carrot than they do in eating cake. They do not think, "I'm fat." (Even though most are!) Babies learn judgments as they grow older. You learned judgment. When you were a child you may have been bribed with food in exchange for compliance. If you complied then you got a sweet treat and a parental stamp-of-approval. But if you defied, you were told that you don't deserve the experience of food-pleasure. Chances are that if you're the defiant type, you probably found a way to get a treat anyway.

I was born defiant so I intimately understand the inner workings of rebellion. No one can tell me what to do! I'll eat my treat no matter what. Two boxes of cookies—that's how defiance plays out. But, none of this represents reality. Whether you got the treat for being good or you stole the treat because you were bad, it doesn't matter because you are actually neither good nor bad—you are a just a human experiencing your body. It's up to you how you want your experience to go. It's true that you don't have control over the events in your life. But you do have control over how you experience those events through your thoughts and actions. I'm talking about your mind-body connection.

The mind-body connection is not as mystic as it sounds. It simply means connecting your thoughts and desires to your actions. But what if you don't like your thoughts or desires? Does connecting your mind and body mean eating two pounds of chocolate is alright because you wanted to? Nope. While you may feel a desire for candy, your body does not really want or need candy. I'm talking about your body, not your tongue. I know you're tongue thinks it wants candy. But how does the rest of your body feel about the effects of that food choice? Mind-body connection is a two-way street between understanding what's deeply rooted beneath your desires and understanding your body's needs. Let me explain. On the surface, you may feel like you have a desire for candy. But really, if you ask yourself deeper questions you'll likely discover that you are trying to meet a need with candy. It's not the candy you want, rather it's what the candy means to you. It's how you feel when you eat the candy. That's what you're really after. You're hooked on a feeling.

Sometimes cravings occur to fill an unmet emotional need. It's common for children to learn that sweet treats equate to happy times. As an adult, sweet treats may be your default mode when you crave happiness. The most peaceful time in my childhood was in the morning when my mother and father drank their coffee. When I feel the need for peace, I usually crave coffee. But, it's not healthy for me to drink coffee past noon or I'm up all night. Because I choose to respect my body, I find non-food related ways to pacify myself when I'm feeling hectic. For example, taking a bath is a peaceful substitute for coffee. And when it's not practical to be naked in water for 20 minutes, I have a go-to song on my phone that provides me with quickie dose of peace—like a mini meditation.

I've had many clients crave crunchy snacks at work. But what they were really craving was some crunch, pop and excitement to break up the monotony and boredom in their day. If you can identify how you're feeling and how you want to feel, then you can devise a plan to create that feeling without eating. So if you're bored at work and you're craving excitement, crank up your favorite jams and dance your ass off for ten minutes! Or plan to test drive some expensive cars at lunch. Put on your favorite red lipstick and a pair of stilettos. Do something that creates the feeling you desire. Get the feeling—fill the void, but not with food.

Sometimes we eat to create a feeling. Other times we eat to avoid, escape or to create a distraction from what we're feeling. For example, when your mind wanders into the past, emotions of resentment, regret, shame, guilt and grief are common. Other times your mind may fear the future with questions like, what if, what then, and how will I? Fear of the future is characterized by feelings of worry, anxiety, anxiousness, nervousness, panic, hopelessness or just being overwhelmed.

Most of us have been through tough times. And who wouldn't be apprehensive to face a coming life challenge? It can feel easier to avoid painful emotions by any means (including emotional eating) rather than facing them. Here's the deal, emotion is energy. In physics, the law of conservation of energy states that energy can neither be created nor destroyed, it can only change form. What I'm saying is that there is no such thing as avoiding your emotions—your emotions will not simply disappear—your emotions may shape-shift, morph or be funneled into another form. The channel you choose for your emotional expression can either facilitate healing or help you avoid or cope.

If you choose food as a coping mechanism, little by little you will eat yourself into another problem. In addition to harrowed emotions, you will also have an unhealthy body. Food only soothes you for a short time.

Afterwards, you are left with a body that feels sluggish, overstuffed and mentally foggy and a mind that feels out of control, full of self-disgust and shame. Don't underestimate the support and stability that a strong, healthy, energetic body can provide you with during tough times.

You may already understand why emotional eating doesn't make sense. That's why they call it emotional-eating and not logical-eating. Our emotional experiences often don't make sense. That's why I don't want you to overanalyze and fight with yourself to end emotional eating. This is not a how-to drop your baggage book. We all have it—baggage is human. Accept it. Love it. It's uniquely yours. It is part of what makes you, you.

Instead of ending emotional eating, begin respectful eating. Honor your body, mind and spirit—quirky baggage and all. You are an invaluable asset to the world. No one can do what you do, the way you do it. There is a reason you are here in this world. And you can't do what you do without your body. So quit hiding your body and your brilliance. Celebrate the fact that you've been to body-war and back. Your food baby stretch marks, scars and sagged out boobs are proof that your body is fighting for you no matter what you do or how you feed it. Unconditionally adapting to get you through. Celebrate your body's incredible loyalty to you at every meal with honorable food choices.

SACRED MEAL TIMES LEADS TO RESPECTFUL EATING

Without understanding why, I became semi-obsessed with purchasing exotic china, crystal and silverware. I ended up hosting my own mini royal dinners, even if it was just a table for one. Every meal was an occasion to drink from my crystal and eat off of an adorned plate. I didn't realize it at the time but I was setting the scene to make every meal sacred. In my home, I require manners at mealtime. Elbows off the table. Sit up straight. Use the right fork and all manner of respectful formality. When you think of a formal dinner you might imagine a stiff no-fun scene. But that's not how my nightly dinner parties roll out. My formality is more about sacredness than proper posture, although that may happen naturally. Manners are a formed habit. Like any habit, at first training yourself to behave with formal dinner manners requires effort, but after a while it becomes second nature—it becomes a habit. I encourage you to eat as many of your meals as possible using a special place setting to signify (to yourself) that eating is an important time to nourish yourself, your mind and your body. Treating meals as sacred naturally leads to respectful eating.

SAY GRACE OR THANK YOU

Resetting your mind is what it takes to begin respectful eating. A great way to set the tone of a meal is by setting an intention to honor what you have and how you receive it. Saying grace, a blessing or giving thanks means acknowledging and feeling grateful for the gift you were given from the higher power (God, Universe, The Divine), in this case the gift is food.

Let me begin by offering a radical idea: grace should precede every meal regardless of its nutritional status. I don't care if you're about to eat an entire cake by yourself in one sitting. Say grace. Get in the habit of inviting your food to the dinner party. Invite your meal into your body for a greater purpose. *Your* greater purpose. Instead of eating with a greedy or unhealthy mindset, eat in gratitude. Instead of asking with entitlement, "What is this food going to give me?" Ask with appreciation for what you have access to, "What can I give or contribute to the world with the energy I receive from this food?" Habitually training your mind to be grateful and training your body to express it by saying grace will reset your attitude towards eating.

Habitually doing or thinking anything with consistency and intention can reset the way you think, feel and act. You get to choose how you connect your mind with your body. Here's how it works. Your brain has billions of cells, called neurons, that have to connect to each other to learn something new including: new behaviors, perceptions and new ways of thinking and feeling. The connections can grow stronger with use or weaker when not used. Habits are the result of particularly strong, frequently reinforced connections—sometimes a connection can grow so strong that it results in automatic behaviors. But you're not doomed to keep thinking, feeling or behaving from your default mode. You can choose to set a new habit or default mode because your brain is reprogrammable, it's called neuroplasticity. Neuroscience research shows us that gratitude, fear, happiness and other states of mind are pathways in the brain that are subject to neuroplastic changes. This means we get to choose our perceptions as well as our behaviors. You can rewire your brain to perceive your body as sexy! You can rewire your brain to get excited about healthy food! You have control over your mind-body connection. The it's-the-way-I-am excuse is out of fashion. Neuroplasticity is in!

I know it can feel daunting to reprogram the way your brain associates emotion with food. I grew up in New Orleans where every day is a special occasion for something sugary, gluten laden or intoxicating. The New Orleans culture worships food like a god. The way I grew up, there are designated foods for every emotion. Eat for joy. Eat for sorrow. Eat for comfort. Eat to get wild. And then there's Mardi Gras. An entire festival devoted to 'eating-up' before you give-it-up. Mardi Gras is a last call for revelry before the Catholic Season of Lent, a time of sacrifice before Easter which traditionally involves giving something up, often a favorite food, treat or indulgence. The mentality of Mardi Gras isn't so different from a diet mentality. It's based on the fear of losing pleasure. The fear of losing pleasure can also extend towards the fear of losing the pleasure you share (connection) with your friends and family over food.

YOU NEED A HEALTHY PEP-SQUAD

It's so easy to be healthy when your social circle is doing the healthy thing. When all the cool kids are eating healthy and exercising, it's easy to follow suit. But, when all the cool kids are encouraging you to cheat, your commitment is tested.

"Come on what's one glass of wine going to do?"
"You've got to live a little!"
"Do you think you're going to live to be 100?"
"You already look great, you don't need to obsess over what you look like."

Here's the rough part, your friends and family want what's best for you, but they probably don't know what's best for you. Friends and family also have their own emotional attachments to food. So when you announce that you're on The Food Baby Detox, they may feel vicariously threatened. Their resistance to your self-improvement has nothing to do with you. They have human perceptions just like you. Maybe they perceive your changes as a suggestion that they should change to. Maybe they don't want to change. Or maybe they do want to change and they just don't have the courage to do it yet. You can probably remember a time when you didn't want to or weren't ready to change. At that time you weren't wrong for being resistant to change and you're not right for being ready in this moment—you were just at a different point in your life. One of the core principles of The Food Baby Detox is self-acceptance. When you empathize and accept yourself, you are more likely to extend that same compassion to others.

The best way to keep yourself in the social loop is to adopt the attitude that The Food Baby Detox is right for you. Accept where your family and friends are and don't allow food to become the focus of your relationship with them. This is a great time to remember why you love the people in your life. It's not because of food. Identify the qualities that endear you to your loved ones. If your relationship has been food-centered or about drinking, think outside of the box and encourage new activities that you can share together. Take a knitting class together. Go to the shooting range and blow up some zombie targets. Have a monthly paint-ball date. Your friends and family will notice when you experience dramatic increases in energy, you lose your food baby, food cravings go away, your sex life sky rockets and you radiate happiness. Live by example. The worst thing you can do is try to convince them to do what you're doing. You may turn them off from health and create disconnection in your relationship, maybe forever. Do not snub their choices. Do not herald your choices. How you feed your body is a personal choice and it doesn't make you good or bad. How your friends and family feed their bodies is a personal choice and it doesn't make them good or bad.

GET OTHERS INVOLVED

Life is always sweeter with support and camaraderie from like-minded people. Invite your family, friends and co-workers to try The Food Baby Detox with you. Notice I said invite not nag. With an open heart and no attachment to whether your invitation is accepted say, "Hey, I'm sick of having a body shape that I don't love. I'm frustrated with being tired and having cravings control my food choices. I want to get healthy and feel proud of my body and my choices. Do you feel any of those things? Would you be willing to experiment with making healthier choices with me?" The worst thing that can happen is they respond with a no. In that case, be totally cool and focus on what you do have in common. The best case is, "hell yes!"

There is incredible power in surrounding yourself with people on the same journey even if it's just for a periodic meeting of the minds. That's why I suggest sharing your journal insights with your food baby bothered friends as a way to stay accountable, support each other and have a high time doing it. It also helps reprogram your mental construct for what good times mean—just as you were programmed to equate good-times with cake at your birthday, you can create new feelings of what good times with good friends mean to you while getting healthy on The Food Baby Detox.

THE UNDER FIVE RULE FOR SIMPLE & QUICK COOKING

My make-it-happen strategy is cooking in bulk, which means cooking about 6 meals at a time. The reason for this is that there is no additional effort required in cooking more of the same. The amount of dishes you dirty is the same—use a larger skillet or pot. I realize this may initially sound like you have to run your own catering company on top of your day job but this is not as bad as it may sound. I created a weeknight standard for cooking and preparing meals called the 'Under Five Rule.' This rule states that no meal shall contain more than five ingredients and shall not require excessive chopping, dicing or slicing. I feel like I need every extra second I can get. I'm sure you do to. Don't get me wrong, I appreciate intricate recipes. Sometimes it's meditative to chop, dice and slice. I also value the ritual of cooking and connecting with your food. Alas, I'm not home for every (okay most) meals and I'm sure you're not either. Pre-preparing your food is the key to making healthy choices easier for on-the-go people. My client's top excuse for not eating healthy is not-enough-time, too busy or I'm never home. This is exactly why coolers and food storage containers were created. Having your meals with you at all times is incredibly freeing because you can keep your schedule open and stay up-for-anything without the stress of locating healthy food or the regret of eating out. If more time and health is what you're after, this is a great solution.

JUST COOK MORE OF THE SAME

The time it takes during your day to order, wait-on and pick up lunch is the same time you'll spend bulk-cooking and packaging five meals. Each day or for five consecutive meals you can (but don't have to) eat the same foods. For me, I start my food rotation (Meal 1) at dinnertime. I cook dinner plus my on-the-go meals for the next day. After the food has cooled, I package my meals for the next day as part of my nighttime cleanup. The next day I just grab and go.

RINSE AND REPEAT—FOOD STORAGE

I prefer not to have an entire day's worth of dishes when I walk through the door at night. That would amount to about ten food containers a day for my family! Therefore, my make-it-happen strategy for my daytime meals is to prepackage my food in parchment paper. If it's a juicy meal that might drip, I slip the parchment paper package into a zipper-lock bag. I realize this isn't the most-green option but it's also not the least-green option. Zipper-lock bags are very compact as opposed to plastic containers that many local health grocers package pre-prepared food in. Of course, I'm not discouraging the use of reusable containers that is clearly the best and greenest option. I'm simply annihilating excuses. If you do use reusable containers, be sure to use glass and not plastic. And never-ever heat your food in plastic. Heated plastics leach synthetic estrogen-like compounds that have been implicated in reproductive dysfunctions in both men and women, cancer and hormonal imbalance. Additionally, do not put your food directly into a zipper-lock bag. Use the parchment paper to provide a barrier between the food and the plastic.

As I suggested earlier, every effort should be made to make mealtime sacred, regardless of where you are. Therefore, I always pack a real fork and a real plate in my cooler. I rarely ever use plastic, it cheapens my food experience.

BE A SOURCE OF FITSPIRATION

It's common for me to have lunch meetings. First I'll tell you what I do, followed by a more socially acceptable suggestion. Sometimes, I eat before going out to eat. At the restaurant I'll order something small and that is certain to be free of the Top Eight foods, like a side salad. Lunch meetings are for talking anyway, right? On days when I'm feeling nonpartisan, I order my side salad and dump my parchment paper-packed meat on top. No one cares. Some people take notes. Own who you are and have confidence in what you do. The results are visual. Everyone will see why you do what you do. You might become someone's fitspiration. If that's too cut-loose for you, most restaurants can grill you a chicken breast or a piece of fish. Order a hamburger or sandwich—hold the bread. Order steamed veggies, baked potato or a side salad and you are good to go!

An empty cooler at the end of the day means that I lived in nutritional alignment with what I want for myself. That feels good. The value in carrying your food everywhere is that you never get caught unprepared. Up-for-anything. Anytime. Anywhere. That's freedom!

My breakfast is simply dinner from the night before, Meal 2 on my rotation. Breakfast doesn't have to be this way. If you are really opposed to having dinner for breakfast, you can make a protein powder shake using one of my four rotatable breakfast recipes. If you do not eat leftover dinner for breakfast, I would strongly recommend eating a dinner-styled meal with an animal protein three to four hours after breakfast. That means if you eat breakfast at seven, you should eat a dinner-styled meal by 10 o'clock.

HAPPY COOKING WITH THE UNDER FIVE RULE

Breakfast Shake-Up

1 TBS nut butter can be added to any shake. Be sure to use a variety of nut butters such as almond butter, cashew butter, pecan butter etc. Almond or coconut milk can be used interchangeably or substituted for water.

Kale Colada

1/2 cup kale
1/4 cup pineapple
1 scoop protein powder (Rotate pea or hemp)
1/4 cup almond or coconut milk
A handful of ice cubes
Sweeten with a touch of honey

Cherry Garcia

1/4 cup cherries (frozen)
1/4 banana (frozen)
1 TBS cocoa powder
2 TBS chia seeds
1/2 cup almond or coconut milk
1 scoop protein powder

Berry Green

3 strawberries
1/8 cup blackberries
1/2 cup spinach
1 scoop protein powder
Optional: almond or coconut milk

Breakfast Bowl

1/3 cup Quinoa
1/2 cup Spinach
4 ounces Chicken
1-2 TBS Nut butter or chopped nuts (almond, cashew, pecan)
Sea Salt to taste

Protein Pancakes

2 TBS Protein Powder (Rotate pea or hemp)
1 tsp coconut butter
1 tsp cacao nibs
1 TBS Nut butter on top (Rotate almond, cashew, pecan)

Protein Oatmeal

1/3 cup cooked Gluten-free oatmeal (use a 1:3 ratio oatmeal:water)
1 TBS Protein Powder (Rotate rice, pea or hemp)
1 TBS coconut oil or ghee
Honey to taste
Cinnamon to taste

Dinner Style Meals for Food Rotation

These meals stay aligned with my core principles of simplicity, quick preparation and tastiness. The style of these meals also makes it easy to serve each family member based on their unique individual nutritional needs. You could very easily serve someone with a high need for protein at the same time as serving someone with a high need for carbs. The ratios of protein, fat and carbs can change for any recipe by adding more of less of each ingredient. These recipes are intended to be cooked with a 'give-a-little, take-a-little' mindset. Just throw in the ingredients in whatever quantities suit you. I've given you a starting point for the amounts of each ingredient—but the true beauty of these recipes is that you cannot mess them up! Below you'll find six different meals you can eat during The Food Baby Detox.

There are 2 possible scenarios for each recipe.
1. Mush it, mix it and put it in a bowl.
2. Put it on a plate.

Chicken

1 Serving
1 Chicken Breast (or 2-3 chicken thighs)
1/2 cup Spinach
2 TBS Almond Butter
1/2 cup Cooked Quinoa
Salt to taste.
Cook the chicken in a large skillet using ghee (clarified butter) or coconut oil on medium heat. Add spinach and allow to wilt.
Optional Spices: Rosemary. Sea Salt Flakes. Pepper.
Mush it + Mix it: Dice the chicken. Add rest of the ingredients.
or
Plate it: Spread nut butter over the top of the chicken. Layer spinach on top of chicken like an open face (bread-free) sandwich. Side of quinoa.

Rice Dressing

1 Serving
2-3 pounds Grass-fed ground Beef, Buffalo or Lamb
1 bunch Green onions, chopped
1/2-1 clove Garlic, chopped
1/2-1 cup Rice
1/4 cup Pecans
Optional Ingredients: bell pepper, celery, eggplant, okra, black pepper.
Cook the ground meat, green onions and garlic in a skillet. Drain the excess fat. Serve over rice and crumble pecans on top. Salt to taste.

Fish n' Chip

2-3 pounds of any variety of fish
1-2 cups Brussels sprouts, purple cabbage or broccoli
Beet chips (sliced thin, salted and dehydrated on 130° for 8-12 hours, see below)
Olive oil or vinaigrette dressing
Optional Spices: cayenne pepper, garlic.
Cook fish, brussels sprouts or broccoli in ghee (clarified butter) on skillet. Pour 1-2 tablespoons of oil on top. Serve with beet chips.

Venison

2lbs venison (meat, liver or hearts)
1 TBS vinegar
1 medium onion
1 cup kale
3 red potatoes
Optional Spices: cumin, pepper, salt
In a large bowl: Marinate meat with vinegar and spices for 1-3 hours. Bake the red potatoes on 350° for 1 hour, then dice. Combine all ingredients in a skillet and sauté with ghee over medium heat.

Pork:

4-5 Pork chops
1 cup Cabbage, shredded
1/4 cup Sesame seeds
Sweet Potato shreds
Olive oil
Optional Spices: fennel, turmeric, chili powder, coriander
Sauté pork chops in a skillet in ghee (clarified butter) over medium heat. Combine with the rest of the ingredients and add 1-2 tablespoons of olive oil on top.

Shrimp

2 pounds Wild-caught shrimp
2 Cucumber
2 Avocado
1 Tomato
1 Mango
2 tablespoons Coconut oil
Sauté shrimp in a skillet in coconut oil until cooked. Chill shrimp in freezer until cool. In a bowl: Add chilled shrimp and the rest of the cold ingredients, diced.
*Fried Option: Dip shrimp into a bowl of melted coconut oil. Then dust in coconut flour. Sauté over medium high heat in coconut oil until golden brown.

Cauliflower Pizza

1 head of cauliflower
1 TBS chopped parsley
1/2 tsp garlic
1/2 tsp oregano
2 TBS arrowroot

1 tsp olive oil

Steam or boil cauliflower until a fork easily pierces it. Place cauliflower into a food processor or blender. Process until mushy. Add the rest of the ingredients and mix. Lay mixture onto a baking sheet lined with parchment paper. Bake at 450° for 12-15.

Pizza Toppings

Sliced tomatoes or tomato sauce
Spinach
Black Olives
Pepperoni (hormone and nitrite-free)

Lower oven temperature to 300°. Layer the toppings onto the cooked pizza crust and bake for another 5 minutes.

When in doubt, keep it simple. A slab of meat with a touch of seasoning, a side of greens and a handful of dehydrated sweet potato shreds (recipe below) is a great default meal that takes no more than 15 minutes to cook.

This list of greens is not all-inclusive it's just a jump-starter for when you draw-a-blank!

Green Vegatable List:

Artichoke	Dandelions	Arugula
Endive	Bok choy	Kale
Broccoli	Lettuce (all kinds)	Brussels sprouts
Mustard Greens	Cabbage	Okra
Celery	Spinach	Chard
Turnip greens	Collard greens	Watercress

Snacks and Treats

Always put your snacks and treats on a plate, sit down and give your body and your food—your attention. Remember: just a dab, will do ya!

Sweet Potato Shreds

Shred sweet potatoes with a vegetable slicer on the shred setting. Sprinkle with cinnamon and salt. Place in a dehydrator or a baking sheet layered with parchment paper. Cook at 130° for 6 hours.

Beet Chips

Slice thinly with a vegetable slicer. Toss in a light mixture of coconut oil or olive oil, salt and dill. Place in a dehydrator or a baking sheet layered with parchment paper. Cook at 130° for 8-10 hours.

Kale Chips

Make absolutely certain the leaves are dry before beginning. Cut the leaves off of the ribs (the stem part) of the kale. Toss in a light olive oil and salt mixture. Line the kale on a baking sheet or dehydrator. Cook at 300° for 6-12 minutes. Check it after 5 minutes—it can go from 0 to done in 30 seconds!

Okra

Toss in a light mixture of olive oil or ghee and salt. Place in a dehydrator or a baking sheet layered with parchment paper. Cook at 130° for 10 hours.

Blueberry-Cacao Crunch

Blueberries

Cacao nibs
Shredded coconut
Coconut milk
Mix all ingredients in a bowl and eat it like cereal!
Optional: add some stevia or honey for sweet.

Coconut Milkshake

1/2 cup whole fat coconut milk
1 tsp vanilla bean powder
3 TBS maple syrup
1 TBS cocoa powder (optional)
1/2 banana (optional)
handful of ice
Place all ingredients in a blender.

Frozen Coffee

1 cup of coffee
2 tablespoons of cacao powder or 1/4 tsp organic vanilla bean powder
or extract
1/2 cup of almond or coconut milk
1 tablespoon of coconut oil
Optional: mint, honey, maple syrup, coconut sugar. A dab will do ya!
Ice
Place all ingredients in a blender.

Jerky

Slice beef brisket or salmon thin. Lightly cover in olive oil, salt, paprika, garlic powder. Line on parchment paper on a baking sheet or place in a dehydrator. Cook at 130° for 12 hours.

Nuts—Any Kind

Soak nuts in a large bowl filled with water overnight. Drain water. Combine 4 cups of nuts in a large bowl with 2TBS ghee (clarified butter), 1TBS salt, 2TBS honey. Spread nuts on a parchment paper lined baking sheet or place in dehydrator. Cook at 150° for 8-10 hours.

Macaroons

3 cups shredded coconut
1/2 cup coconut butter
3 TBS coconut flour
2 TBS vanilla extract
1/3 cup of cacao nibs (optional)
1/4 tsp salt
Mix all ingredients in a large bowl. Squeeze and make small balls about 1/2 inch in diameter. Place on a parchment paper lined baking sheet. Cook at 250° for 45 minutes.

Fried Bananas

Slice bananas, fry in coconut oil over low-medium heat for five minutes until the color changes and it develops a mushy consistency. Mush and serve in a bowl. Optional: dip bananas in coconut flour for a more authentic fried treat!

Almond Butter Cookies

2 cups of almond butter
1/2 tsp vanilla extract
3 TBS of coconut flour or arrowroot
1/4 cup applesauce
1/4 cup cacao nibs (optional)
Mix all ingredients. Make small balls. Place on parchment paper lined

baking sheet. Bake at 350° for 10-12 minutes.

HAPPY PANTRY

Most people do best when the only options available are healthy ones. Some people can keep treats in the house and use them appropriately. But I'm not that girl. Out of sight, out of mind is more like my motto. Even a nice healthy piece of organic dark chocolate doesn't last long in my pantry. If you can stay aligned with your goals and keep treats in the pantry then go for it. Otherwise stick to The Food Baby Detox basic staples.

My happy-pantry stash recommendations:

Acai powder	Coconut milk	Almond flour
Coconut shreds	Almond milk	Dehydrated Okra
Camu Powder	Gluten-free oats	Chia seeds
Jerky	Cocoa flour	Nuts
Cocoa nibs	Quinoa	Coconut flakes
Rice		

Oils: ghee (clarified butter), coconut butter, coconut oil, olive oil.

In the freezer:

Frozen asparagus	Frozen spinach	Frozen berries
Frozen prepared meals for on-the-go		

CHALLENGE MEALS

At the end of The Food Baby Detox, you will need to reintroduce one food (soy, gluten, dairy, eggs, corn and legumes) at a time for up to four days for each one. Refer to Chapter 5 for the complete list of details regarding how to conduct this self-experiment. Below you'll find a few of my favorite, very healthy challenge recipes.

Challenge Eggs: Quiche Muffins

Makes approximately 12 regular sized muffins or 6 oversized muffins
5 eggs
1/2 cup almond milk
1 lb cooked ground meat of your choice (turkey, chicken, beef, pork or diced shrimp)
1/2 cup of chopped broccoli
2 TBS chopped parsley

Whip eggs in a bowl. Add the rest of the ingredients. Lightly spray muffin tins with a coconut oil spray and pour mixture into the tins. Bake at 350° for 25 minutes or until the tops are lightly browned.

Challenge Corn: Southern Belle Grits

Makes approximately 5 meals
1 cup yellow grits (unprocessed)
2 TBS of ghee
3 cups of water or almond milk
1 lb cooked meat (diced chicken or shrimp is best)
1/4 cup chopped green onions or shallots as we call them down South.
Sea salt and pepper to taste

In a large pot, combine all ingredients. Cook on medium heat for 10 minutes or until the water is absorbed and the consistency is viscous. Stir occasionally.

Challenge Soy: Miso Soup

Makes 1 serving
Purchase miso at your local grocer. It comes in a little tub-like container in the cold section.
Add 3 TBS of miso to 3/4 cup of boiling water. Stir and enjoy!

Challenge Dairy: Cheesecake

Makes 10 servings

Nut Crust

1 cup of nuts (almonds, pecans, hazelnuts)
1/2 cup (1 stick) real butter!
1 cup of arrowroot
1/8 cup of stevia, coconut sugar or date sugar (1/4 cup for those who like things sweeter)
1/4 sea salt
1/2 teaspoon vanilla extract

Place nuts in food processor, process until the consistency is composed of very fine bits. Add remaining ingredients and process until smooth. Press mixture into a lightly buttered baking dish or pie plate. Bake at 350 for 20-25 minutes.

Cheesecake

24 oz cream cheese
1/8 cup real milk
1 TBS vanilla
3/4 cup stevia, coconut sugar or date sugar

Let cream cheese soften to room temperature. Mix with stevia, coconut flour and vanilla. Beat until creamy and smooth. Poor over cooked nut crust. Bake in oven at 325 for 50 minutes. Turn oven off and let sit for another 10 minutes before removing.

Cheesecake is best if left to refrigerate for 24-36 hours. So hard to do, but worth the wait!

Challenge Legumes: Red Beans and Rice

1 pound red kidney beans (soaked overnight and drained)
1/2 cup diced onions
1/2 cup diced celery
1/2 cup diced green bell pepper
2 TBS parsley
2 TBS minced garlic
1 TBS sea salt
1/2 tsp cayenne pepper
1 lb sausage and diced ham chunks
7 cups water

In a large pot sauté all ingredients except the red beans. Add red beans and water to the mixture. Cover the pot and cook on low heat for 5 hours or until soft and creamy. Serve over rice.

Using my Under Five Rule, cook it with just kidney beans, sausage, salt, cayenne and rice.

chapter seven

SELF-REFLECTIVE JOURNAL

———

• Describe your relationship with food. Eat to live or live to eat?

• Do you use food to distract yourself or create a feeling you desire? Give an example of what you're thinking or feeling while you eat.

• How can you create the feelings you desire without food? For example, if you desire comfort and peace — you can take a hot bath and listen to music? Make a list of feelings that you have been creating with food and then give one example of how you can meet your need without food.

• Were you ever bribed, rewarded or punished with food as a child?

• How do you bribe, reward or punish yourself as an adult?

• How do you plan to continue The Food Baby Detox as a way of life? Name 3 action items that you commit to maintaining a healthy lifestyle and your plan for how you will make it happen. For example, "I will cook and pre-package my food for the next day — every night while listening to great music."

LISTENING TO YOUR
BODY IS TIMELESS

———

I'm a world-class information junkie and I frequently suffer from fact overindulgence. Sometimes, I have to consciously unplug from reading the latest and greatest research because my whirring mind tries to override my inner voice and my body's communication to me. New research will continue to reveal the complexities of the human body. New discoveries will be made and there will always be a new diet to experiment with. The beauty of The Food Baby Detox is that new research can't invalidate this process of self-discovery to connect you closer to the inner wisdom of your body. Mind-body connection. The proof is in your response to the pudding. Go with your gut and trust that when symptoms of food baby bloating, fatigue, skin problems, food cravings and low sex drive improve, you are on your right path. Listening to your body is timeless. I hope you'll join me and other emboldened seekers to continue on the self-discovery path at nikidriscoll.com.

Wishing you self-love and happiness,

Niki

RECOMMENDED READING AND RESOURCES

---

www.nikidriscoll.com/foodbabydetoxsupplements

www.kristencampbellbeauty.com

Adrenal Fatigue: The 21st Century Stress Syndrome
James Wilson and Jonathan V Wright

Biochemical Individuality
Roger Williams

A Course In Weight Loss: 21 Spiritual Lessons in Surrendering Your Weight Forever
Marianne Williamson

A-Z Guide to Drug-Herb-Vitamin Interactions
Health Notes Inc., Alan Gaby MD, Steve Austin, Forrest Batz, Eric Yarnell, Donald Brown, Donald Brown, George Constantine

Eat Fat, Lose Fat
Mary Enig and Sally Fallon

Food Allergies and Food Intolerance: The Complete Guide to Their Identification and Treatment
Jonathon Brostoff and Linda Gamlin

How to Eat, Move and Be Healthy
Paul Chek

Metabolic Typing Diet
William L. Wolcott

Nourishing Traditions: The Cookbook That Challenges Politically Correct Nutrition
and the Diet Dictocrats
Sally Fallon

Nutrition and Physical Degeneration
Weston A. Price and Price-Pottenger Nutrition Foundation

Your Body's Many Cries for Water
Fereydoon Batmanghelidj
The Yoga of Eating: Transcending Diets and Dogma to Nourish the Natural Self
Charles Eisenstein

Your Hidden Food Allergies Are Making You Fat
by Roger Deutsch and Rudy Rivera M.D.

BIBLIOGRAPHY

Agreus L et al.The epidemiology of abdominal symptoms: prevalence and demographic characteristics in a Swedish adult population. A report from the Abdominal Symptom Study. Scand J Gastroenterol 29 (1994): 102-109

Alvarez WC. Hysterical type of nongaseous abdominal bloating. Archives of Internal Medicine (JAMA). 84:217–45 (1949).

Baumgart DC, Dignass AU. "Intestinal barrier function." Current Opinion in Clinical Nutrition and Metabolic Care. 5(6) (November 2002):685-94.

Biesiekierski JR, et al. No Effects of Gluten in Patients With Self-Reported Non-Celiac Gluten Sensitivity After Dietary Reduction of Fermentable, Poorly Absorbed, Short-Chain Carbohydrates. Gasteroenterology. 145(2):320-328 (August 2013).

Bijkerk CJ, Muris JW, Knottnerus JA, et al. Systematic review: the role of different types of fibre in the treatment of irritable bowel syndrome. Alimentary Pharmacology Therapy. 19:245–51 (2004).

Bizzaro N., et al. Cutting-edge issues in celiac disease and in gluten intolerance. Clinical Review of Allergy Immunology. 42(3) (June 2012):279-87.

Bjarnason I, Takeuchi K. "Intestinal permeability in the pathogenesis of NSAID-induced enteropathy." Journal of Gastroenterology. 44(19) (2009): 23–9.

Brown K, et al. Diet-Induced Dysbiosis of the Intestinal Microbiota and the Effects on Immunity and Disease. American Journal of Gastroenterology. 109(2014):741–746.

Casazza, K., et al. "Myths, Presumptions, and Facts about Obesity." New England Journal of Medicine 368 (2013):446-454.

Catassi C. The global village of celiac disease. Recenti. Progressi in Medicina. 92(7–8) (2001): 446–450.

Connell J.M., et al. Effects of ACTH and cortisol administration on blood pressure, electrolyte metabolism, atrial natriuretic peptide and renal function in normal man. Journal of Hypertension. 5(4):425-33 (August 1987).

Corazziari, E. Definition and epidemiology of functional gastrointestinal disorders. Best Practice and Research Clinical Gastroenterology. 18(2004):613-31.

Den Hartog G., et al.The constipated stomach. An underdiagnosed problem in patients with abdominal pain? Scandinavian Journal of Gastroenterology. 225(1998):41-6.

Discovery's Edge, Mayo Clinic's Online Research Magazine. Celiac Disease: On The Rise, July 2010

Drossman D., et al. Householder survey of functional gastrointestinal disorders. Digestive Disease and Sciences. 38(9): 1569-1580 (September 1993).

Drossman DA. Chronic functional abdominal pain. American Journal of Gastroenterology. 91(11):2270-81 (November 1996).

Drossman, D.A., et al. U. S. Householder survey of functional gastrointestinal disorders. Digestive Diseases and Sciences. 9(38) (September 1993): 1569-1580
Eggesbu M, Halvorsen R, Tambs K, Botten G. Prevalence of parentally perceived adverse reactions to food in young children. Allergy Immunology. 10(122) (1999): 132

Fass R. "Functional heartburn: what it is and how to treat it." Gastrointestinal Endoscopy Clinics of North America. 19 (1): 23–33 (January 2009).

Garzon DL., Kempker T., Piel P. Primary Care management of food allergy and food intolerance. The Nurse Practitioner. 36(12) (2011): 34-40.

Gasbarrini G., et al. Origin of celiac disease: How old are predisposing haplotypes? World Journal of Gastroenterology. 18(37):5300-5304 (2012).

Gibson AR, Clancy RL. "An Australian exclusion diet". Medical Journal of Australia. 1 (5) (March 1978): 290–2.

Gibson PR, Shepherd SJ. Evidence-based dietary management of functional gastrointestinal symptoms: The FODMAP approach. Journal of Gastroenterology and Hepatology. 25(2):252-8 (February 2010).

Grammar K., et al. Darwinian aesthetics: sexual selection and the biology of beauty. Biological Review. Cambridge Philosophical Society. 78(2003): 385-407.

Gyires K Tóth ÉV Zádori SZ. Gut inflammation: current update on pathophysiology, molecular mechanism and pharmacological treatment modalities. Current Pharmaceutical Design. 20(7):1063-81 (2014).

Houghton LA, Whorwell PJ. Towards a better understanding of abdominal bloating and distension in functional gastrointestinal disorders. Neurogastroenterology and Motility. 17:500–11 (2005).

Huang J., Chaloupka F.J., Fong G.T. Cigarette graphic warning labels and smoking prevalence in Canada: a critical examination and reformulation of the FDA regulatory impact analysis. Tobacco Control. 23(1):i7-12 (March 2014).

Jiang, X., et al. Prevalence and risk factors for abdominal bloating and visible distention. A population based study. Gut (BMJ Group) 57 (2008): 756-63.

Jones HW, Jones GS. Pelvic pain and dysmenorrhea. In: Berek JS, Adashi EY, Hillard PA, eds. Novak's Textbook of Gynecology. 12th ed. Baltimore, Md: Williams & Wilkins; 399-428 (1996).

Kabbani TA, et al. Celiac Disease or Non Celiac Gluten Sensitivity? An Approach to Clinical Differential Diagnosis. American Journal of Gastroenterology. 109(2014):741–746.

Kasarda, D. Can an Increase in Celiac Disease Be Attributed to an Increase in the Gluten Content of Wheat as a Consequence of Wheat Breeding? Journal of Agricultural and Food Chemistry. 61(6):1155-1159 (February 2013).

Leffler DA et al. The interaction between eating disorders and celiac disease: an exploration of 10 cases. European Journal of Gastroenterology and Hepatology. 19(3):251-5 (2007).

Lembo, T., Naliboff, B., Munakata, J., et al. Symptoms and visceral perception in patients with pain-predominant irritable bowel syndrome. American Journal of Gastroenterolgoy. 94(1999):1320–6.

Lenoir M., Serre F., Cantin L., Ahmed S.H. Intense Sweetness Surpasses Cocaine Reward. PLoS ONE 2:e698 (2007).

Lewis MJ, Reilly B, Houghton LA, et al. Ambulatory abdominal inductance plethysmography: towards objective assessment of abdominal distension in irritable bowel syndrome. Gut(BMJ Group). 48(2001):216–20.

Lohi S, Mustalahti K, Kaukinen K et al. Increasing prevalence of coeliac disease over time. Alimentary Pharmacology and Therapeutics. 26(9) (2007):1217–1225.

Longstreth, G.F., et al. Functional Bowel Disorders. Gastroenterology 130 (2006):1480-1491.

Malik VS., et al. Sugar-sweetened beverages and weight gain in children and adults: a systematic review and meta-analysis. American Journal of Clinical Nutrition. 98(4):1084-102 (October 1998).

Maxton DG, Morris JA, Whorwell PJ. Ranking of symptoms by patients with the irritable bowel syndrome. British Medical Journal. 299 (1989):1138.

Montalto M, Santoro L, D'Onofrio F et al. "Adverse reactions to food: allergies and intolerances." Digestive Disease 26 (2)(2008): 96–103.

Mustalahti K, Catassi C, Reunanen A et al. Coeliac EU Cluster, Project Epidemiology. The prevalence of celiac disease in Europe: results of a centralized, international mass screening project. Annals of Medicine. 42(8), 587–595 (2010).

National Institutes of Health, U.S. Department of Health and Human Services. Opportunities and Challenges in Digestive Diseases Research: Recommendations of the National Commission on Digestive Diseases. Bethesda, MD: National Institutes of Health. (2009) NIH Publication 08–6514.

Niestijl Jansen, J. et al. Prevalence of food allergy and intolerance in the adult Dutch population. Journal of Allergy and Clinical Immunology. 93(2) (February 1994):446-56.

Plaks & K. Stecher. Unexpected improvement, decline, and stasis: A prediction confidence perspective on achievement success and failure. Journal of Personality and Social Psychology. 93:667-684 (2007).

Reilly BP, Bolton MP, Lewis MJ, et al. A device for 24 hour ambulatory monitoring of abdominal girth using inductive plethysmography. Physiological Measurement. 23:661–70 (2002).

Rubio-Tapia A., et al. Increased Prevalence and Mortality in Undiagnosed Celiac Disease. Gastroenterology. 137(1):88–93 (July 2009).

Sanchez, A., et al. Role of Sugars in Human Neutrophilic Phagocytosis, American Journal of Clinical Nutrition. 261:1180-1184 (Nov 1973).

Schmulson, M., Lee, O.Y., Chang, L., et al. Symptom differences in moderate to severe IBS patients based on predominant bowel habit. American Journal of Gastroenterology.

94(1999):2929–35.

Seo,, Y., Kim, N., Hyun Oh, D. Abdominal Bloating: Pathophysiology and Treatment. Journal of Neurogastroenterology and Motility. 19(4): 433-453 (2013).

Shatenstein S, et al. Eliminating nicotine in cigarettes. Tobacco Control. 8(1):106-109 (March 1999).
Singh D. "Adaptive significance of female physical attractiveness: role of waist-to-hip ratio". Journal of Personality and Social Psychology. 65(2): 293–307 (August 1993).

Skoog SM, Bharucha AE. Dietary fructose and gastrointestinal symptoms: a review. American Journal Gastroenterology. 99:2046–50 (2004).

Song JY, Merskey H, Sullivan S, et al. Anxiety and depression in patients with abdominal bloating. Canadian Journal of Psychiatry. 38:475–9 (1993).

Swagerty DL Jr, Walling AD, Klein RM. Lactose intolerance. American Family Physician. 65:1845-1850 (2002).

Talhout R, Opperhuizen A, Van Amersterdam JG. Sugars as tobacco ingredient: Effects on mainstream smoke composition. Food and Chemical Toxicology. 44(11):1789-98 (2006 Nov).

Talley NJ, Dennis EH, Schettler-Duncan VA, et al. Overlapping upper and lower gastrointestinal symptoms in irritable bowel syndrome patients with constipation or diarrhea. American Journal of Gastroenterology. 98:2454–9 (2003).

Thompson WG, Longstreth GF, Drossman DA, et al. Functional bowel disorders and functional abdominal pain. Gut. 45(2):43-7 (September 1999).

Thompson WG, Longstreth GF, Drossman DA, et al. Functional bowel disorders and functional abdominal pain. Rome II. Functional Gastrointestinal Disorders: Diagnosis, Pathophysiology, and Treatment. second edition. Degnon Associates, Inc; Mclean, VA: 2000. pp. 351–432.

Tomiyama A.J., et al. Low calorie dieting increases cortisol. Psychosomatic Medicine. 72(4):357-64 (May 2010).

Van der Hulst, et al. Glutamine and the preservation of gut integrity. The Lancet. 341(8857):1363-1365 (May 1993).

Vos MB, et al. Dietary fructose consumption among US children and adults: the Third National Health and Nutrition Examination Survey. Medscape Journal of Medicine. 10(7):160 (July 2008).

Wadley G, Martin, A. Origins of agriculture: a biological perspective and a new hypothesis. Australian Biologist 6: 96-105 (June 1993).

Yoshida Y, Sasaki G, Goto S, Yanagiya S, Takashina K. "Studies on the etiology of milk intolerance in Japanese adults". Gastroenterology Japan. 10 (1): 29–34 (1975).

Yoshikawa T, et al. Association of fatigue with emotional-eating behavior and the response to mental stress in food intake in a young adult population. Behavioral Medicine. 40(4):149-53 (2014).

Young, E., et al. A population study of food intolerance. Lancet. 342(8906) (May 1994):1127-30.

Yucel B et al. Eating disorders and celiac disease: a case report. International Journal of Eating Disorders. 39(6):530-2 (2006).

ABOUT THE AUTHOR

Niki Driscoll is a speaker, writer and health coach specializing in teaching the mind-body connection. She merges the latest happiness research with nutrition and exercise science—to help you discover an authentic, fulfilling and joyful way to eat, move and live. Her motto is listen to your body, follow your heart and take your brain with you! Niki has been in private practice for over 15 years coaching clients in holistic health and natural remedies, personal training and rehabilitation, massage therapy, nutrition and life coaching. Visit nikidriscoll.com for tips on the psychology and spirituality of eating, exercise and body image.

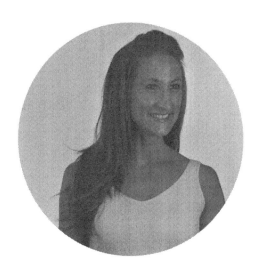

INDEX

5-HTP, 137

A

abdominal bloating, 1, 3, 6, 7–8, 12, 175, 177, 180
abdominal fat, 6, 12, 43–44, 138
abdominal pain, functional, 180
abdominals, 37, 51, 55
Abdominal Symptom, 175
absorption, 88, 134
acne, 18, 48, 83, 134, 135
adaptogenic, 137
addiction, physical, 68, 69
addictive qualities, 78
adrenal gland, 41, 52
age, 23, 24, 77, 80, 135, 155
alcohol, 11, 34, 37, 57, 75, 78
allergies, 18, 29, 31, 58, 179
Allicin, 134
almond oil, 139, 140
almonds, 89, 114, 119, 156, 157, 164, 167
American Journal of Gastroenterology, 175, 176, 178, 179, 180
amino acids, 75, 97, 98, 136, 138
ancestors, 77, 94
animal protein, 98, 156
anti-inflammatory properties, 132, 134, 138, 139

antimicrobial, 137, 138
anti-nutrients, 78, 87, 88
antioxidants, 84, 135, 137
antiperspirants, 58
appearance, 28, 36, 68, 129, 130
apples, 89, 101, 114, 119
arrowroot, 79, 114, 165, 167
artichoke, 114, 117, 119
artificial sugars, 22, 64, 66, 67, 76, 111, 120, 122, 132
Artificial Sweetener, 36, 66–67, 69
asparagus, 114, 117, 119
aspartame, 67
attitude, 11, 121, 150, 152
avocado, 114, 116, 160

B

bacteria, 32, 33, 48, 78, 81–82, 131, 132
  friendly, 32, 75, 111, 132, 135, 140
bacterial ratios, 32, 33–34, 69, 99
baked goods, 84, 87, 89
balance, 50, 72, 73, 82, 83, 99, 101
beans, 87, 114
  red, 168
beauty, 10, 12, 158, 171, 177
beef, 99, 113, 116, 119, 166
beer, 36–37
behavior, 102, 151

Made in the USA
Middletown, DE
09 July 2016